Stigma and Social Support on the Supplemental Nutrition Assistance Program

Stigma and Social Support on the Supplemental Nutrition Assistance Program

Laura Blount Carper

LEXINGTON BOOKS
Lanham • Boulder • New York • London

Published by Lexington Books
An imprint of The Rowman & Littlefield Publishing Group, Inc.
4501 Forbes Boulevard, Suite 200, Lanham, Maryland 20706
www.rowman.com

86-90 Paul Street, London EC2A 4NE

Copyright © 2022 by The Rowman & Littlefield Publishing Group, Inc.

All rights reserved. No part of this book may be reproduced in any form or by any electronic or mechanical means, including information storage and retrieval systems, without written permission from the publisher, except by a reviewer who may quote passages in a review.

British Library Cataloguing in Publication Information Available

Library of Congress Cataloging-in-Publication Data Available

ISBN 9781793655189 (cloth : alk. paper)
ISBN 9781793655202 (pbk. : alk. paper)
ISBN 9781793655196 (electronic)

♾️™ The paper used in this publication meets the minimum requirements of American National Standard for Information Sciences—Permanence of Paper for Printed Library Materials, ANSI/NISO Z39.48-1992.

Contents

List of Figures and Tables   vii
Acknowledgments   ix

1	My Experiences with SNAP	1
2	Factors Influencing SNAP Enrollment	11
3	Bringing Everything Together: Theory Application	33
4	Summary of Study Findings	49
5	General Views of SNAP Themes	65
6	Stigma and SNAP Enrollment	75
7	Disclosing SNAP Enrollment Concerns	99
8	Social Support from Family and Friends and SNAP Enrollment	119
9	Factors That Influence Enrollment and Implications from Findings	131

Appendix A: Factor Analysis   141
Appendix B: Past and Present Methodology   145
Appendix C: Survey Demographics   153
Appendix D: Interview Schedule   155
Appendix E: Procedure and Intercoder Reliability in Interview Data   157
Appendix F: Limitations   159

Appendix G: Survey Instrument	161
Bibliography	167
Index	175
About the Author	181

List of Figures and Tables

FIGURES

Figure 2.1　Bronfenbrenner's Social Ecological Systems Theory and Independent Variables　13
Figure 4.1　The Predicted Probabilities for Total Stigma, Past Consequences Stigma, Anticipated Consequences Stigma, and SES Stigma (IV) and Enrollment Status (DV)　55
Figure 7.1　Concern for Disclosing SNAP Enrollment to a Specific Person Examples　114

TABLES

Table 4.1　Demographic Characteristics of Participants in Survey　53
Table 4.2　Themes from Interviews Code Book　60
Table 6.1　Hierarchical Logistic Regression Results for Total Stigma (IV) and Enrollment Status (DV)　77
Table 7.1　Hierarchical Logistic Regression Results for Past Consequence from Disclosing SNAP Enrollment Stigma (DISC-12, IV) and Enrollment Status (DV)　101
Table 7.2　Hierarchical Logistic Regression Results for Anticipated Consequences from Disclosing SNAP Enrollment Stigma (DISC-12, IV) and Enrollment Status (DV)　104
Table 7.3　Hierarchical Logistic Regression Results for Concern for Disclosing SNAP Enrollment to a Specific Person (Wright et al., IV) and Enrollment Status (DV)　108

Acknowledgments

This book was made possible by the many individuals who have had stigmatizing experiences on SNAP; these individuals are the reason why I love working on projects that hopefully will provide benefit to further generations of participants who use SNAP.

Through this process I appreciate the guidance, advice, editing, statistics help, and so on, of my advisors Dr. Loretta Pecchioni, Dr. Renee Edwards, Dr. James Garand, and Dr. Catherine Moon who have all been so helpful and understanding throughout the entire process, and I am forever grateful for everything they have done. For Dr. Pecchioni, I have appreciated our long chats about family and life in COVID-19 and helping me to narrow down the mountain of a project that I started out with. Dr. Renee and Dr. Garand have provided not only great help with statistics but also a great ear to listen to many of life's problems. Meeting and establishing a rapport with Dr. Catherine Moon is a highlight of this process.

My amazing and large family is the reason I am here today. I am forever grateful to my mom Rebecca Blount, dad Crandall Blount Sr., and siblings Marnita, Corissa, and Crandall Blount Jr. who have taught and sacrificed their time to take care of my children when I needed to write and take classes. Their love and support for me over the many years of continued education will forever be empowering for me.

If anyone deserves a section in the acknowledgment, she is my grandmother, Tinita Blount. For many years she has been a role model for me. She is headstrong, empowering, loving, and stubborn. She has always pushed me in my endeavors and encouraged me that I could do more. I am so thankful for hours she has spent editing, providing advice, and keeping me on track throughout this process. She is my inspiration.

I am forever thankful for my extended family including Forrest and Arlene Carper, and Wesley, Carlene, and Liliana Martin for their support and love throughout the process. I am forever grateful for the support of my church family, which includes many who have been there for me in the process from the beginning being my guinea pigs from early development of the surveys to the end. They provided many laughs and comments such as "Laura, I feel like you are interrogating me." One more friend requires a shout-out—Rebekah Whitaker. From the start, Rebekah has been there for me at LSU providing friendship and advice. Thank you.

Lastly, my faith in God has helped ease many stressed nights and provided me peace and direction in life. Without his guiding hand, I would not be where I am; my faith will always be an important part of my life.

I dedicate this book to my personal family who have sacrificed throughout this process: my precious Robert, Alaina, and Winston Carper. You are my world!

Chapter 1

My Experiences with SNAP

Through many years of research, my personal experiences with SNAP and other welfare programs have shaped my research focus in health and risk communication. To not discuss my personal experiences with SNAP would be leaving out a crucial piece of my field of research. A description of my reasons for enrolling, experiences on the programs, and observations of others on welfare inform my interest in these issues and may also bias my interpretations. I hope the reader finds that my experiences are reinforced by the reports of others' experiences and agrees that the stigma associated with needing assistance should be reduced.

REASONS FOR ENROLLING

In May 2013, I was finishing up my undergraduate degree at Southeastern Louisiana University when my boyfriend (now husband), Robert, and I discovered we were three months pregnant with our daughter Alaina. This was quite a shock for us, as my boyfriend was currently a graduate student studying English and an Airman in the Louisiana Air National Guard, and I was a teller at a local bank. I was diagnosed with hyperemesis gravidarum early on in the pregnancy which is essentially extreme morning sickness. I quit my job at the bank and pushed back my starting date for my master's program until after the birth. We were relying solely on his income, which was based on his GI bill and graduate assistant salary at Southeastern. We applied for SNAP benefits immediately following our marriage in July 2013 and began receiving about $300 (which was increased to $550 following her birth) a month for a total of two years, before my husband was hired in a higher paying job. Furthermore, we were enrolled on Women's, Infants, & Children (WIC) for another year after the birth of our son in 2016. Thus, we were enrolled in a type of welfare program for four years. We debated heavily before enrolling because of the shame we had heard from others about being enrolled and not being able to provide for ourselves.

OUR EXPERIENCES WHILE ENROLLED

The stigma and shame from being enrolled was enforced in our social circles. Some members of our social groups informed us that enrolling was our fault, and that we should have planned better before getting pregnant. Specifically, some of my extended family members were not supportive. The common narrative from extended family was, "We never had to rely on the federal government, and we were poor, too." While we had heard this narrative several times, it became more salient after we enrolled and had accidently told some extended family members about the possibility of enrolling; after being scolded, my husband and I decided to no longer talk about our enrollment on SNAP or WIC with others. Because we felt the need to not disclose our welfare status, we began to feel shame and depression for using it. Both my husband and I felt that we had failed and that our advanced degrees had done nothing to help alleviate our situation. Though we felt guilt and shame for enrollment, we were conflicted, knowing that we needed the program to provide us with healthier food options during my pregnancy and after birth. However, as soon as our financial situation improved, we left both programs.

Some family members, on the other hand, were more supportive/lenient of our SNAP enrollment. My parents had been WIC recipients immediately following my birth in 1992 until 1995 while my father was a welder and my mom a kindergarten teacher. They often described how they knew what we were feeling because of the stigma they had experienced from friends. Having my parents as a possible source of support helped us through the years with our experiences. While there was some stigma and shame from family members, there were some issues with friends as well.

Besides some family stigma from SNAP enrollment, the largest impact on our social circles was losing friendships. Once I left my job, I lost most of my primary sources of friendship and began to feel isolated. My husband had moved from Baton Rouge, and his GA at Southeastern did not lead to many friendships, so neither of us was meeting with or discussing our SNAP membership with others. A few years later when I was doing a study on SNAP enrollment, I disclosed to some of my church friends that I had been enrolled, and they were shocked to know that we had been enrolled. Some even said, "I had no idea you were enrolled; I thought with a better education and your job at the bank that you were fine." They were very supportive, and we had great discussions about our experiences enrolled. However, it is important to note that I was not currently enrolled in SNAP at the time when I disclosed the enrollment. While I was enrolled, I did not want to disclose to any of my church friends or family my enrollment because of social media posts, discussions I heard from others, and experiences at stores.

Then, and especially now, I often see social media posts about "users of the government," "get a job (which we had)," "lazy," "stealing my tax dollars," and so on. These posts depressed my husband and me because we felt that we were grouped in the category and that people viewed us negatively. When we would go to Walmart (especially) and Winn-Dixie, we often heard slurs about the contents of our shopping cart if the person behind us saw us use an EBT/SNAP card or WIC voucher. One time specifically at Walmart, an individual saw me checking out with the EBT/SNAP card while I was very pregnant and commented, "See another user with a Michael Kors purse and pregnant and not working using food stamps." I was so upset, I cried when I got in my vehicle. The Michael Kors purse was actually a Dooney & Burke that my grandmother had gifted me for my 20th birthday. Though it has been several years, I remember this encounter vividly as one of the most stigmatized experiences while enrolled on SNAP. We experienced WIC stigma more often because of the use of the voucher system (thankfully, this has been transferred to cards). We were less likely to experience any negative comments at local grocery stores instead of big chains, so we quit going to Walmart and Winn-Dixie because of the experienced stigma and went to smaller stores until the end of our enrollment.

During our time with SNAP and WIC, we developed a greater respect for individuals on the program and the stigma they are experiencing. I was inspired to conduct research on underprivileged individuals living in poverty because of the often-expressed sentiments of being downtrodden by society and struggling to stay afloat. Though I was only enrolled for a short time and have an element of privilege being a white female, I felt stigma from my enrollment and wanted to know if/how others experienced stigma while they were enrolled. Overall, my enrollment taught me to keep a more open discussion about the world around us and what other people are experiencing, because until one actually experiences something for himself or herself, it often seems like the situation is exaggerated.

INTRODUCTION

My personal experiences have informed my interests in the issues of stigma and social support for individuals who are enrolled in assistance programs; I am interested in learning if others have similar experiences or not. First, stigma are the feelings of shame associated when a person feels he or she does not meet another's standard of behavior (Goffman, 1963). In other words, stigma is a feeling associated with being a "marked" individual by outside groups as a break in a perceived norm. Stigmas are very important when considering how SNAP enrollment may make the participant feel poorly as described in my experiences. I will further describe the different elements of stigma which will be included in a later chapter. Besides my experiences with stigma, I also discuss in my experience with the SNAP program the importance of positive social support. Because social support is the social interaction with others with the goal of providing actual or at least perceived support to a person, positive social support is considered a factor that reduces stress and improves mental health (Harandi et al., 2017). Both stigma and social support are important social determinants of health that will be discussed further; however, before addressing stigma and social support, basic information about these programs is essential because misinformation or lack of information about them often helps to fuel misconceptions about their use, qualifications for enrollment, and how individuals experience being enrolled.

THE IMPORTANCE OF SNAP

The SNAP is a federal assistance program that provides income to purchase food. To be eligible for the program, one's yearly income must fall below 130% of the poverty line; in 2019, this translates to $32,640 for a family of four (United States Department of Agriculture [USDA], 2019). As of July 2020, 38 million individuals in the United States receive SNAP benefits, with an average $136.36 per person, while 19.5 million households receive an average of $266.86 (USDA, 2020). In the "Characteristics of the SNAP households: Fiscal year 2019" of the individuals enrolled, 35.7% are Caucasian, 25.1% are African-American, 16.7% are Hispanic, 3.0% are Asian, and the remaining are Native American, multiple races, or not disclosed (USDA, 2019). Research has found that SNAP enrollment helps reduce food insecurity and poverty (Gregory & Deb, 2015; Yen et al., 2008) and improves overall health. In 2018, 44.2 million Americans or 14% of the U.S. population received benefits and the number was continuing to increase (United States Department of Agriculture [USDA], 2018). Food insecurity is a significant predictor of poor health outcomes (Gundersen & Ziliak, 2015), which makes success of the program essential.

The purpose of SNAP is to provide supplemental assistance to low-income families by providing them a monthly allowance to buy nutritional food which otherwise would not have been available (Nestle, 2019). While the guidelines for SNAP have changed over the years, the primary purpose of SNAP is to provide assistance to the poor.

A form of SNAP has existed since the Great Depression of the 1930s as a way to help farmers with their loss of crops, but it was not until the early 1960s that a pilot version of what is today's SNAP program was created under the Johnson administration (Roth, 2015). The SNAP program was created to increase the food-buying power of low-income people, allowing them access to more nutritious foods. In 1977, the Food Stamp Act was passed allowing individuals entitled to support if they met eligibility requirements.

The Food Stamp Act was changed in 2009 to the SNAP to facilitate the idea that a name change was needed to provide healthier options to participants than "food stamps" previously allowed (Cucurullo, 2012). Even with the name change, SNAP is often the subject of debate by lawmakers arguing that the current stipulations (participants can currently purchase many items such as soda, candy, chips, and other fatty foods) allow for more unhealthy food options and result in higher levels of obesity in children compared with those who are not on the program. Although it has been argued that SNAP causes higher consumption of fat and sugar which can lead to obesity (Jensen & Wilde, 2010), Kinsey et al. (2019) suggested that SNAP has effectively reduced poverty and food insecurity for low-income families.

In addition to SNAP, in times of weather-related events, such as floods and hurricanes, the federal government can issue the Disaster Supplemental Nutrition Assistance Program (D-SNAP). D-SNAP has different requirements from SNAP. Individuals who are not normally enrolled in SNAP could apply for benefits if they have a business or home damaged by the disaster, lost food or supplies, lost a job or have reduced work hours, and so on ("D-SNAP," 2019). Individuals who are already on SNAP would then have additional funds added to their account using D-SNAP. The D-SNAP and SNAP programs may provide a unique perspective into the different stigma elements of both programs.

Though not a specific element of SNAP, multigenerational poverty may increase enrollment on SNAP. In addition to the impacts on poverty of individuals, there is research that indicates poverty may be multigenerational. Herbert Gans (2011) describes how poverty is often seen as a temporary time in one's life; some people remain poor for many years and may have been from families and prior generations that have also been poor. Thus, multigenerational poverty is a poverty that has occurred for several generations in one family. Gans argues that multigenerational poverty is likely not insignificant because "America still contains a number of sub-regional 'pockets of poverty' as well as poor rural communities, small towns, and urban neighborhoods that have been poor for a long time" (p. 71). He further proposes that there are five main areas associated with multigenerational poverty: hereditary and transmitted disease and similar capacities, poverty-related situational crises (such as poor-performing schools), vulnerabilities (face more problems but have fewer tools to be able to deal with problems when they arise), racial and class factors, and coping patterns. Of the five, the most pertinent to SNAP stigma and social support is how multigenerational poverty is linked to race and class. Specifically, Gans (2011) states,

> Many of the country's multigenerational poor are from African-American and other nonwhite populations. Racial stigmatization, discrimination, and segregation not only are continuing obstacles for the nonwhite poor but also continue to shackle future generations. (p. 76)

Because of the impacts of multigenerational poverty, I believe it is important to analyze the multigenerational use of SNAP to determine how individuals who have had multiple generations enrolled on SNAP may feel differently about the program than individuals who are first-generation SNAP users. Generational SNAP usage will not analyze multigeneration poverty exactly because families may have qualified for SNAP but chose to not enroll.

Considering the breadth and history of the program, there are many possible factors that may influence enrollment. According to a report by Keith-Jennings and Chaudhry (2018), the length of time enrolled on SNAP differs per the circumstance. Participants can receive SNAP until they lose eligibility, or participants can be members for temporary assistance. The USDA states that half of all participants leave SNAP within one year, and two-thirds leave within two years. Those who participate the longest tend to be people who are older or people with disabilities. While the report says two-thirds of all SNAP participants leave after two years, no details are provided to describe why people leave or their experiences while enrolled. Individuals who are older and have disabilities may enroll longer on SNAP because of long-standing issues that continue to limit their income, whereas individuals that are enrolled shorter amounts of time may have more temporary circumstances (such as looking for a new job or medically unable to work). However, I am interested in seeing if the stigma from being enrolled on SNAP may also influence leaving the program earlier. If people are leaving the program partly because of the stigma from being enrolled, I am interested in changing the rhetoric of the way people talk about the program in regards to who is eligible. In Keith-Jennings and Chaudry (2018), no background is given on the demographics of a person who is likely to leave. Because of the importance of SNAP on overall health of impoverished individuals, I believe there is value in determining what experiences while enrolled could lead someone to choose to not enroll any longer. Furthermore, there is a need to determine what the differences are between an individual that is currently enrolled and one who is no longer enrolled. There may be many differences present between current and past participants such as different viewpoints of stigma—possibly an individual may choose to leave the program because of stigma or a change in employment and remember that stigma differently from individuals who are currently enrolled and experience the stigma daily. Because I think that individuals who are no longer enrolled may remember their stigmatizing experiences differently from those individuals who are currently enrolled where the stigma is more salient and current, I will be operationalizing enrollment in SNAP as those individuals who are currently enrolled and those that are no longer enrolled. Furthermore, I will also be comparing current and past members to determine if stigma and disclosure concerns are different between these two groups. Understanding what influences enrollment on SNAP is essential for improving the usefulness of the program to individuals to increase the advantages of being enrolled.

SOCIAL DETERMINANTS OF HEALTH AND THE ECOLOGICAL MODEL

I have provided a suggested framework to help identify and focus the number of possible variables. Because so many factors may come into play when determining impacts to enrollment, one possible way to examine and narrow down the many possible impacts to SNAP enrollment is to apply Bronfenbrenner's ecological model to analyze demographic variables that are also social determinants of health. The ecological model arranges all of the different contexts of development into five levels of influence. The individual's factors are then affected by the immediate physical and social environment (microsystem); interactions between systems and the environment (mesosystems); broader social, political, and economic conditions (ecosystem); larger general beliefs and attitudes shared by members of the society (macro-systems); and the chronosystem or life events that impact individuals over the life span (Bronfenbrenner, 1979). The social determinants of health can then be placed into the different levels. The social determinants of health, according to the World Health Organization, are,

> The circumstances in which people are born, grow up in, live, work, and age. This also includes the systems in place to offer health care and services to a community. These circumstances are in turn shaped by a wider set of forces: economics, social policies, and politics. ("Social determinants of health," 2008)

Social determinants of health include income inequality, educational opportunities, occupation and employment status, gender inequity, racial segregation, social support, experienced stigma and discrimination, and immigration (Lehmann, 2019). While many social determinants of health may impact SNAP enrollment, I primarily focus on the communication about stigmatizing experiences on SNAP as well as the social support provided when discussing these experiences. Stigma and social support provided on SNAP have been analyzed in several studies which found the program has had many negative consequences on a person's well-being, including felt stigma and shame (Vancil, 2008; Smith, 2007; Fricke et al., 2015). Though not heavily researched, in general, applying communicative theories to understanding the reasons why individuals consider leaving SNAP will help indicate how stigma (a socially constructed concept) is communicated through conversation and the importance of social support and coping with that stigma. Most importantly, my research will help provide policy makers with better information about the negative aspects of SNAP as a whole, and possibly identify larger societal issues as well. In addition to social support and stigma, some other social determinants of health (which are essentially demographic variables)—income, education, gender, race, and immigration—will be included to examine any possible interactions with social support and stigma. The ecological model will then be used to describe how elements such as migrant status, age, immigration status, educational attainment, and gender are micro-level elements, whereas stigma, race, and social support span many different levels. Providing these levels will help organize the breadth of variables into more useable pieces of information. Though I will be using demographic variables that are examples of social determinants of health, I will not be analyzing how these variables impact overall health or the success of the SNAP program as a whole on overall health; I am interested in how negative stigmatized experiences on SNAP are communicated to others and are influenced by the different levels of the ecological model and in turn impact one's enrollment.

I have discussed the importance of SNAP enrollment and how using demographic variables that are also social determinants of health is an option to provide a more structured framework to analyze the difference across members enrolled in SNAP currently and in the future. I will now briefly describe the theoretical focus of my study. Even though SNAP impacts a large number of disadvantaged and often stigmatized individuals, very little research has been done to analyze the population in general, but even fewer in the field of communication studies. To better understand how stigma and social support impact enrollment on SNAP, the results will be grounded in Bronfenbrenner's (1979) ecological systems theory which proposes multiple, interlocking levels. In particular, I will be examining specific points in the individual, micro, and meso levels with some elements possibly crossing into the macro-level and chronosystem. Although I will not be analyzing any specific points that may address larger general beliefs and attitudes about SNAP (macrosystem) or life events that impact individuals over their life span (chronosystem), the findings of the second part of the study may cross into these levels. Additionally, I will apply different stigma theories and concepts—including Charles Horton Cooley's "looking glass self-theory," and Erving Goffman's "spoiled identity"—to help describe the impacts of stigma on one's personal identity. To help bring context to the abundance of information from the interviews, narrative theory, Relational Dialectics and the chain of discourses, and the Communication Management Privacy theory will be applied to determine how social support and stigma on SNAP enrollment exists in relationships, stories, and privacy management in Chapter 3. While none of these theories has been applied to SNAP research, I believe these theories can help frame and explain the factors that influence enrollment on SNAP.

I am providing a mixed-methods design study that analyzes the impacts of variables—specifically social support and stigma—on SNAP enrollment. Chapter 4 provides the results of a survey instrument constructed to include a variety of stigma measures and the previously identified social determinants of health (demographic variables) to determine if there are differences between current and past recipients of SNAP. Chapter 6 will include the elements of stigma that were found to be statistically significant in Chapter 4, then develop into an interview schedule to discuss how current or past SNAP participants talk about the significant stigma variables with members of their social circles and determine what, if any, social support is provided. Now, I will describe in further detail possible factors that may influence SNAP enrollment and how to organize them.

Chapter 2

Factors Influencing SNAP Enrollment

Considering the breadth and history of the program, there are many possible factors that may influence enrollment. One possible way to help describe how variables may impact SNAP enrollment would be to use Bronfenbrenner's social ecological theory and apply factors that are social determinants of health because I am using populations that are living in poverty and face many of these determinants daily. First, to explain why I have chosen to include demographic variables that are also social determinants of health, I will provide a brief discussion of how people who are enrolled on SNAP could also be experiencing some health disparities which are connected to social determinants of health. According to the National Institutes of Health, health disparities are health differences among different groups of people and can include race, gender or sex, immigrant status, geography, sexual orientation, and income (National Institute of Health [NIH], 2016). The social determinants of health and health disparities can help describe why differences exist across members of several groups. The social determinants of health are helpful because these demographic variables help define why health disparities occur in many underprivileged communities.

One specific way in which I can analyze experiences on SNAP is to look at the intersectionality of multiple groups. Intersectionality, a concept first defined by Crenshaw (1989), is the idea that social group membership such as gender, race, and class does not exist in a vacuum, but that an individual can be a member of multiple groups. Since I am interested in stigma and social support, I will need to attempt to tease out the intersectionality of these various statuses with being a SNAP recipient which indicates an individual who lives in or on the edge of poverty. Participants of SNAP are members of possibly multiple underprivileged groups including racial differences, gender, different levels of education, and immigration/migrant status as well as being impoverished. All of the variables are examples of social determinants of health. The social determinants of health may provide a helpful established framework to help organize and narrow down demographic variables of individuals who are living in poverty (and have possibly come from many generations of poverty) and enrolled in SNAP. As a reminder, though health disparities and the social determinants of health are primarily used to measure overall health of an individual, the demographic variables used in the current study will serve as a way to organize, not to measure, overall health or to analyze the effectiveness of SNAP. To further describe how the social determinants of health—racial differences, educational attainment, immigration/migrant status, gender, and so on—the social ecological model can then be used to determine how these factors may influence one's view of the SNAP program.

THE SOCIAL ECOLOGICAL MODEL

Overall, Bronfenbrenner's social ecological systems theory frames the first phase of this study. As mentioned earlier, social ecological models help to organize factors that influence and affect behavior and to develop programs through inclusion of the social environment. Social ecological models include multiple levels of influence depending on the behaviors being analyzed. Urie Bronfenbrenner initially postulated the social ecological models in the 1970s and 1980s to better understand the complex process of human development. He suggests that an individual's inherent qualities and environments do influence how the person grows and develops in life (Bronfenbrenner, 1979). The ecological model arranges all of the different contexts of development into five levels of influence. The individual's factors, such as gender and migrant status, are then affected by the immediate physical and social environment (microsystem); interactions between systems and the environment (mesosystems); broader social, political, and economic conditions (ecosystem); larger general beliefs and attitudes shared by members of the society (macrosystems); and the chronosystem or life events that impact individuals over the life span (Bronfenbrenner, 1979).

Using Bronfenbrenner's model, I situate my primary variables of stigma and social support, as well as race, gender, education, age, and immigrant status, as seen in figure 2.1. Individual factors may include, but are not limited to, migrant status, age, educational attainment, immigration/migrant status, and gender, whereas stigma, race, and social support span several layers and may even impact individuals throughout their life span.

Bronfenbrenner's model will help organize the variables into a more manageable model to highlight how stigma and social support may be impacted

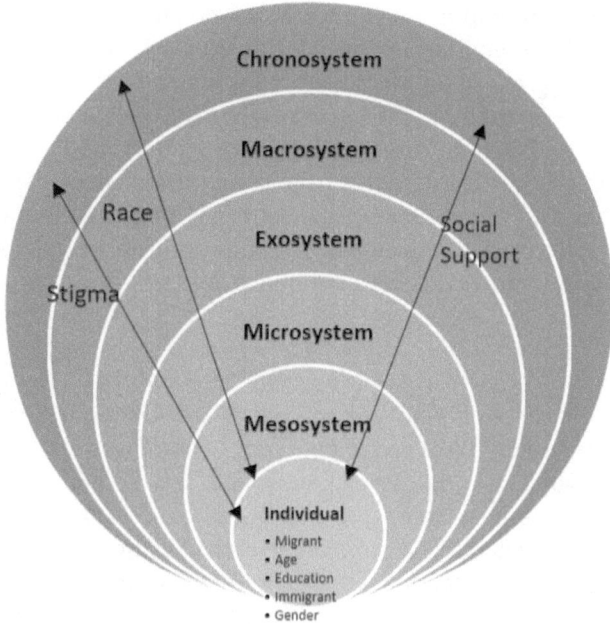

Figure 2.1 Bronfenbrenner's Social Ecological Systems Theory and Independent Variables. *Source:* Created by the author.

at different levels of social interaction for an individual enrolled in SNAP. Please note that while I understand many other factors that are larger or public-scale problems that may impact SNAP enrollment, I will focus on more individual factors which may influence enrollment on SNAP, including how individuals interpret larger-scale factors within their circumstances. To help describe further, Louisiana (where I am from) provides a unique opportunity to analyze how the social determinants of health (demographic variables) may impact SNAP enrollment.

LOUISIANA AND SNAP ENROLLMENT

As I was conducting my study, I primarily focused on Louisiana citizens because I received benefits in Louisiana, I currently reside in Louisiana with my family, and staggering amounts of poverty exist in the state. Louisiana has some of the highest numbers of per capita SNAP enrollment in the United States. According to the World Population Review (2020), Louisiana ranked second in the country with the number of people per capita enrolled in SNAP. In Louisiana, 17% of the population is enrolled in SNAP or roughly 810,000 individuals. Furthermore, 71% of SNAP participants are families and children, 37% are in families with members who are elderly or disabled, and 39% are in working families (Nchako & Cai, 2020). Louisiana is consistently ranked in the top five states with the highest amount of poverty (19.6% of the population), according to the United States Census Bureau (2019). While Louisiana has a history of larger numbers of individuals living in poverty when compared to different areas of the country, Louisiana also provides a unique sample with a presence of diverse racial and ethnic communities in several parishes, issues in education, and the use of immigrant and migrant workers in agricultural and construction jobs.

Race

In addition to the amount of poverty in Louisiana, there are several parishes in which minority groups make up the majority. According to the USDA (2017), 82.6% of the population in New Orleans and West Baton Rouge (District 2) is African American compared to 13.3% Caucasian. The Shreveport, Bossier City, and Natchitoches area population (District 4) is 61.1% African American and 35.3% Caucasian. Lastly, District 5, or the Monroe/Alexandria area, population is 60.4 African American with 37.8 Caucasian population. Overall, of the six districts in Louisiana, half have Black or African American population making the majority of the population, which is especially important compared to the overall racial breakdown in Louisiana with 62.9% Caucasian, 32.7% African American or Black, 1.8% Asian descent, and 5.2% Hispanic or Latinx ("Profile of SNAP household," 2017).

In comparison, the overall racial breakdown of SNAP participants in the United States, according to the USDA (2013), reports 40.2% are white, 25.7% African American, 10.3% Hispanic, and 2.1% Asian. Now that I have provided data that indicates a unique racial dynamic in regards to SNAP enrollment, I will suggest how Louisiana can provide a sample of migrant workers.

Migrant Status

Migrant status for my current study will include individuals who are here on working visas such as the H-2A or H-2B or work only temporary jobs. Migrants are an understudied population experiencing disparities in health; Dilberto et al. (2018) suggested that temporary migrants send a larger proportion of their payback home with the intention of returning home at some point. Furthermore, temporary migrants are less likely to bring family members when they come to work, meaning they are lacking very crucial social support. While migrants are lacking the necessary social support in their daily lives, they are also experiencing stigma and discrimination and lack the aid to cope with this stigma. According to the United Nations (2019), migrants are listed as a vulnerable group to racism. As a vulnerable population, migrants experience severe discrimination in housing, education, health, work, and social security because of a rise in xenophobia (racist sentiment and discriminatory practice). Importantly, many migrants also live in poverty. In addition to those who work as a migrant or temporary worker, immigrants face similar challenges. The Center for Immigration Studies (2010) found that 43.6% of immigrants lived in or near poverty compared to 31.1% of natives. Including migrant workers into the sample of factors that influence SNAP enrollment could provide useful information on a group that is experiencing different types of stigma at one time.

According to U.S. Labor Department's Office of Foreign Labor Certification, Louisiana ranks fifth in the United States for the number of H-2A employments with 7,115 certified agricultural workers. The H-2A is a temporary agricultural program that allows employment in areas where domestic workers are low and the positions need to be filled. Employment with the H-2A is seasonal in nature and lasts no longer than a year ("H-2A certification," 2018). In addition, Louisiana employs 5,147 Latinx individuals who come as H-2B temporary nonagricultural workers. H-2B workers are very similar to H-2A except for the positions being nonagricultural in nature ("H-2B certification," 2018). Please note that H-2A and H-2B migrant workers arrive on visas and are not illegal immigrants, which is beyond the scope of my study but possibly impacts enrollment on SNAP as well. Analyzing migrant status is necessary when interpreting factors that influence enrollment on SNAP. Now that I have discussed poverty, race, and migrant status in Louisiana, I will conclude with education.

Education

According to the U.S. News (2019), 30% of Louisiana's population is college educated with a median income of $28,885 a year. Louisiana is consistently ranked as the state with the most problems in education, but the delivery of education is not what I am concerned with. I am, however, interested in how those who have higher educational attainment experience stigma while enrolled on SNAP and whether their education level impacts their enrollment on SNAP. Today, it is becoming expected that in order to avoid a lower social economic status and poverty, as well as to achieve better overall health, one must attain a higher level of education (beyond high school); however, reality indicates this is sometimes not the case. Shankar et al. (2013) report that minority and indigenous groups in Canada struggle to earn a livable wage with a more advanced degree. In interviews with several individuals with master's and doctoral degrees, Patton (2012) found that individuals having advanced degrees reported frustration from receiving food stamps. One quote from a doctoral student in Florida highlights the frustration and stigma from being highly educated and enrolling in SNAP:

> He says he has taught more than two dozen courses in communications, performing arts, and the humanities, and he has watched academic positions in these fields nearly disappear with budget cuts. When he and Ms. Stegall stepped inside the local WIC office in Tallahassee, Florida, where they used to live, with their children in tow, he had to fight shame, a sense of failure, and the notion that he was not supposed to be there. After all, he grew up in a family that valued hard work and knowledge. His father was a pastor and a humanities professor, and his mother was a psychology professor. (p. 1)

Another comment that also highlights the plight of those with further education is seen by a former adjunct professor–turned consultant, "It's gone beyond the joke of the impoverished grad student to becoming something really dire and urgent," says Ms. Kelsky. "When I was a tenured professor, I had no idea that the Ph.D. was a path to food stamps" (p. 1).

From these two studies, higher education can be associated with less pay or even poverty and enrollment in federal welfare systems. Further research is needed to determine how individuals with higher amounts of education experience stigma as well as social support received for the feelings of inadequacies. While the lack of education is a social determinant of health and is linked to poverty (Waxman, 1976), very little research applies stigma to those who have more education and stigma from SNAP enrollment.

Overall, I have discussed poverty, race, migrant status, and education as possible secondary social determinants of health (demographic variables) that can be used to describe the impacts on enrollment in Louisiana. Because research is lacking in how these demographic variables impact enrollment on SNAP, I am proposing a research question one that will address which demographic variables (that are also social determinants of health—migrant status, immigrant status, race, and education) impact SNAP enrollment.

STIGMA AND SOCIAL SUPPORT

After describing the importance of SNAP, the social determinants of health, and the social ecological model as a framework to provide structure to the numerous factors that may influence enrollment, stigma and social support will be discussed as the primary importance for SNAP participants' experiences.

Stigma

I am proposing that stigma may impact enrollment on SNAP and the social support received. First, I will describe what stigma is, then elements of measuring stigma that could help analyze SNAP participation, and, lastly, I will provide theories that can help ground stigma in communication.

First conceptualized by Goffman (1963), stigmas are the feelings of shame associated when a person feels he or she does not meet another's standard of behavior. In other words, stigma is a feeling associated with being a "marked" individual by outside groups as a break in a perceived norm. Stereotypes are then created as an overgeneralization of a group to attempt to "place" a person in one of these categories and then provide a label or mark to that person. The "mark" of a stigmatized individual is defined by several dimensions of stigma. Jones et al. (1984) describe different dimensions of stigma, including how concealed a particular condition is, the course (does the mark change over time), is the mark disruptive (does it block or hamper communication and interaction), to what extent does the mark make the possessor repellent, ugly, or upsetting (aesthetic qualities), under what circumstances did the condition originate, and what danger does a marked person pose to society. Stigma can then be seen as a socially constructed process in which identification is used to determine which group a person may fit into based on several factors to judge a marked person (Kunreuther & Slovic, 1999). The various dimensions of stigma help to define how these negative attributions are created, labeled, communicated, and reinforced.

Because of these various dimensions and processes, a discussion of research that has defined different types of stigma is necessary.

Types of Stigma

Many different types of stigma have been defined and analyzed in a variety of fields and studies. Herek et al. (2013) described four different types of stigma experienced by people with HIV/AIDS: internalized, felt normative, enacted, and vicarious. Internalized is the stigma that once it is experienced, the person contains and buries it inside instead of dealing/coping with the stigma. Felt normative is when the individual believes the stigma is warranted. For example, if SNAP recipients believe that they are using others, and they feel that other SNAP participants are as well, they may feel that the stigma is warranted. Enacted stigma is defined as actual physical harm being performed on an individual for being a part of the marked group. Lastly, vicarious stigma occurs when one is not experiencing the stigma firsthand but experiencing it through a third party. This third party could be through the use of social media and reading posts to hearing friends talk about others on the program. In other words, the individual is experiencing stigma through the eyes of another, not from a direct interaction with a stigmatizer. I feel there is a need to determine if current and past recipients of SNAP experience these different types of stigma while they are enrolled. The first three hypotheses relate to how current SNAP participants will report higher levels of perceived, internalized, and felt normative stigma, whereas research question 2 explores how vicarious stigma may differ in current and past recipients because of the lack of studies in vicarious stigma and SNAP enrollment. Lastly, hypothesis four postulates that current SNAP participants will experience more total stigma than those who were no longer enrolled. Unfortunately, after the initial factor analysis (which will be further described in appendix A), the different types of stigma become narrowed down in this study into three specific stigma variables: total stigma (chapter 6), and past and anticipated consequences from disclosing SNAP enrollment stigma (chapter 7). Research question 3 then clearly defines how the different types of stigma (generalized SNAP enrollment disclosure concern stigma, past consequences from disclosing SNAP enrollment stigma, and anticipated consequences from disclosing SNAP enrollment stigma) are experienced for current and past recipients of SNAP. In addition to the different types of stigma, I also analyzed how the different types of sources of stigma could also impact enrollment.

Herek et al.'s work helped define experiences of stigma, but Brohan et al. (2013) developed the DISC-12 or the discrimination and stigma scale as a means to determine the differences among sources of stigma. The DISC-12 was created in Great Britain to measure the sources of mental health stigma such as from family, friends, or being poor (2013). DISC-12 can help determine how the different types of stigma can vary by the source of that stigma. Combining both Herek's different types of stigma and DISC-12 sources of stigma will offer a more nuanced view of stigma experienced by individuals on SNAP to provide useable information about the impacts on enrollment.

While Herek's types of stigma and DISC-12 sources of stigma help organize the broad umbrella of stigma research, neither instrument helps describe why stigma can be an impactful experience. The emotional and intrapersonal value of being stigmatized is better described by Goffman's work and Berger et al.'s (2001) work with self-image and other theories in communication.

"Spoiled Identity"

Goffman describes how stigmas can create a sense of personal devaluation for the stigmatized group to the extent that members of the group are no longer considered human. Furthermore, due to being stigmatized, the groups are now discriminated upon by outside members of the group impacting their health. The experienced stigma then impacts the person's own individual identity. Goffman (1963) describes it this way,

> Discrepancy may exist between an individual's virtual and actual identity. This discrepancy, when known about or apparent, spoils his social identity; it has the effect of cutting him off from society and from himself so that he stands as a discredited person facing an unaccepting world. (p. 19)

"Spoiled identity" then impacts how the other persons see themselves and how others see them as well, as seen in this quote:

> When normal and stigmatized do in fact enter one another's immediate presence, especially when they attempt to sustain a joint conversational encounter, ... these moments will be the ones when the causes and effects of stigma must be directly confronted by both sides. The stigmatized individual may find that he feels unsure how we normally will identify him and perceive him. (p. 13)

Goffman is suggesting that how a stigmatized person and the stigmatizer interact is based on how the stigmatized feels about himself, and the interaction may be uncomfortable because of perceived feelings toward the stigmatized.

While the stigmatized are members marked by society for being members of the disadvantaged group, they may also have negative images of themselves. The differences between an individual's "virtual and actual identity" can further be explained by Charles Cooley's "looking glass self" and Higgins's self-discrepancy theory.

"Looking Glass Self" and Self-Discrepancy Theory

Charles Cooley describes the "looking glass self" as a reflection of how we think others view us. Cooley suggests that we use the "looking glass self" in three steps: (1) how one imagines one looks to other people, (2) how one imagines the judgments of others by how they are viewed by the other person, and (3) how a person may view somebody else based on past judgments. In this way, any social interaction is seen as a "looking glass" that allows the person to determine how others may see him or her and form a negative self-esteem (Cooley, 1902). Adding to Cooley's work, Higgins (1987) describes the self-discrepancy theory that self-esteem is determined by how one compares the ideal self (the characteristics he or she wants to possess) and the ought self (the person others wish and expect one to be); when there is a difference between ideal and ought self, one's perception is said to be discrepant and leads to lower self-esteem. An example for applying "spoiled identity," "looking glass self," and self-discrepancy theory is a stigmatized individual on SNAP. If a person feels that being a SNAP recipient is negative from either self or how others view the person, this may go against ought self (I just need to get a better job), causing low self-esteem and eventually leaving the program to save face.

Low self-esteem can also lead to a negative self-image. Berger et al. (2001) developed a scale to measure stigma that includes how stigma creates a negative self-image and causes disclosure concerns. They found that negative self-image relates to feeling bad about oneself having HIV. In other words, Berger suggests that negative feelings can impact one's self-image and can manifest as feelings of guilt or shame. This description implies Herek's definition of internalized stigma.

Smith (2007) found that SNAP recipients feel they are marked members of the "welfare" system. Furthermore, recipients have been researched for years as being stigmatized for not only being poor but also as users of the "welfare" systems. The stigmatization can be further deepened based on being from minority groups, older individuals, stigmatizing health conditions, sexual orientation, and so on. Thus, all of these different stigmas are interacting with each other before one even enrolls in SNAP. Once the person enrolls, the participant is now labeled a "SNAP" or "food stamp" user and may experience perceived, internalized, and felt normative stigma.

Furthermore, Vancil (2008) performed a study that analyzed factors that impacted accepting benefits, meaning the person declined enrolling in SNAP. Vancil's sample from Wisconsin acquired data through interviews and found several themes: people choose not to enroll because of the lack of accessibility to the food stamp program, the stigma associated with the program, bureaucratic issues, the lack of information about the program, and the feeling of not deserving the benefits. I am particularly interested in the different types of stigma associated with the program as well as the feelings of not deserving the benefits, which I believe relates to the impacts of the different types of stigma and enrollment. Though the study does not highlight what types of stigma are present and causing people to decline enrollment, the results are still important to note that individuals perceive the threat of stigma just from enrolling.

In addition to Vancil and Smith, Fricke et al. (2015) found that SNAP participants reported experiencing statements such as "You just want a hand out" negatively impacted how they felt about the program in general, suggesting the individuals could have internalized and perceived the stigma and negatively impacted how they feel about SNAP. Furthermore, depending on the person, individuals may have felt that society was marking them as a user, and then in turn feel they deserve these negative assessments of themselves (felt normative stigma). Because of the research in HIV and stigma scales, as well as Goffman's spoiled identity, the "looking glass self" by Charles Cooley and Smith (2007), Fricke et al. (2015), and Vancil's (2008) studies in SNAP suggest that participants in SNAP deal with stigma on many levels, and this stigma may in turn influence the likelihood to disclose that enrollment to others.

Disclosure Concerns

Berger et al. (2001) and Sayles et al. (2008) suggested that people who are experiencing stigma also have concerns with disclosing their "marked" status to others. Specifically, Berger et al. (2001) found that because of negative experiences with others and having HIV, they had more disclosure concerns relating to keeping their HIV status secret and controlling who knows. In the earlier discussion of Goffman and "spoiled identity," he suggests that those that are stigmatized have trouble disclosing their stigma to others because it is contradictory to how they wish to be viewed and often choose to hide that information (Goffman, 1963). The same results were found by Reinius et al. (2017) where disclosure concerns were defined as "Controlling information, keeping one's HIV status a secret, or worrying that others knew about respondent's HIV status and would tell" (p. 2). Sayles et al. (2008) adapted the Berger scale but included disclosure concerns and found similar results that higher amounts of disclosure concerns led to higher amounts of experienced stigma and shame. Specifically, Sayles et al. add fears, "I am concerned if I go to the HIV clinic, someone I know might see me" or "I am concerned that if am sick, people I know will find out about my HIV." These concerns relate to the idea of spoiled identity and Cooley's looking glass self. The responses suggest the impact of self-image and negative self-identity. Based on the past research in disclosure concerns and stigma, I seek to determine in research question 4 how generalized SNAP enrollment disclosure concerns differ for individuals who are currently enrolled on SNAP and those who are no longer enrolled.

Now that I have discussed what stigma is, the different types of stigma, theories of stigma in communication, and the possibility that stigma may also influence how one discloses SNAP enrollment, I will now define what social support is and its importance in the discussion of stigma and SNAP enrollment.

Social Support

The essential problem with disclosure concerns from SNAP enrollment is the possibility that participants would be unable to receive social support to help them with possible stigma from their enrollment. If a person feels so stigmatized from enrollment, he or she may feel unable or unwilling to reach out to others, possibly leading to issues with overall mental health. Participants may also feel like that because they feel stigmatized; they may not know to whom they should reach out for help about their enrollment. Considering the importance of social support and SNAP enrollment, I will provide an overview of what social support is and why it is so valuable to have in relationships. Uchino (2004) provides a broad definition of social support, stating that it "includes both the structures of an individual's life (for example, group memberships or existence of family ties) and the more explicit function they may serve" (p. 10).

Additionally, Cutrona and Suhr (1992) combined past research in social support to describe five different types of social support: informational, tangible, esteem, emotional, and social network support. Informational support relates to advice given by others. For example, if a SNAP participant learned to enroll on the program from another person to help them enroll. Tangible support is social support given in the form of needs or goods, such as money or food. Esteem support helps promote one's personal skills, worth, and abilities. An individual who is enrolled on SNAP or has been enrolled in SNAP might receive esteem support if someone tells the person, "Do not worry, you will overcome this; you are strong," or "I know you will do good on any future job." Emotional support relates to expressions of care, love, concern, empathy, and sympathy. As related to SNAP, emotional support could look like "I love you no matter, and I am here to help with any needs you might have." Lastly, social network support relates to the feeling of being supported by a group, such as being offered to be a part of a support group.

Next, social support can be enacted or perceived. Enacted support research focuses on the quantity and existence of relationships and on the structure of one's social network, whereas perceived support is the perception that support is there when one needs it (Goldsmith, 2004). Thus, enacted support is what has been received, and perceived support is the knowledge that support is available if needed.

To further define social support, both Uchino (2004) and Vaux (1988) describe the process of social integration or how interconnected the individual is among one's social ties and roles. Social networks research examines the actual social structure as well as the interactions that take place in the network. Important considerations in analyzing social networks are the size of the group, frequency of contact, the content of exchange in relationships, and many others (Vaux, 1988). Furthermore, the social network theory suggests that social structure around a person influences his or her beliefs and behaviors (Liu et al., 2017). For example, Eapen (2016) found that a majority of pregnant women received support from family members, while some help was reported through friends. Immediate family members provided physical support, informational support, financial help, and emotional support during pregnancy and delivery. From friends and coworkers, they primarily received financial and informational support, suggesting the type of social support differs based on the role of the specific person. Research in sociology and health has found that people who are embedded in supportive social ties have better health and better lifestyles (Browning & Cagney, 2002; Mohen et al., 2011; Pinxten & Lievens, 2014). However, not all research has found that social support positively impacts health. In fact, enacted social support can have no effect or a negative effect.

Wellman (1981) suggested that information flows through a person's social networks and such information may or may not be supportive. Not surprisingly, success in providing social support is based on the outcome of the support provided and the costs of that support. Thus, there are times when social support can be appropriate and effective but at different times may be harmful (Goldsmith, 2004). For example, Domínguez and Arford (2010) found that strong social ties promote brain health as one ages, but if a person has obese friends or family, the individual is more likely to be obese. Now that I have described social networks and ties in general, I will provide one example of a study applying social support to SNAP usage.

Korlagunta et al. (2014) analyzed how older adults used SNAP to purchase and prepare food and how social support can affect the likelihood to use SNAP. When the participants became unable to grocery shop and prepare food, social support increased. Furthermore, both family and friend interactions were significant predictors of the ability to grocery shop and prepare food. However, friend interactions had slightly more influence on the likelihood to use SNAP compared to family interactions. Korlagunta et al. (2014) did not address why there was a difference between family and friend interactions, and they did not address any social support received from family or friends.

When applied to my current study, social support, individual networks, and social ties that participants bring with them when they enroll in SNAP may influence their likelihood to stay in the larger SNAP network. To describe why I am using stigma and social support as a means to discuss the stigma of enrollment, I will provide a discussion of studies that have analyzed both stigma and social support together.

Social Support and Stigma Research

Previously, I have provided a discussion of what social support and stigma are, studies applying to SNAP research, and an application of these studies to communication concepts such as "spoiled identity" and "looking glass self"; now I will describe why I chose to analyze both social support and stigma as the primary independent variables (IV) that may impact enrollment on SNAP. Social support and stigma are listed as primary social determinants of health (primary IV), meaning that the amount of social support received is essential to a healthy lifestyle, and the smaller amounts of stigma the better. In fact, reducing stigma correlates with help-seeking behaviors such as increased disclosure, and the more social support received can reduce stigma (Mokkarala et al., 2016). To further describe the impact of social support on stigma, several studies analyzed this relationship.

While large amounts of research in stigma are primarily focused on individuals diagnosed with HIV/AIDS, this is not the case for all studies incorporating both social support and stigma. Topics can range from unintended pregnancy (Moseson et al., 2019), people living with HIV in China (Xiao et al., 2018), and pharmaceutical opioid dependence (Cooper et al., 2018; Birtel et al., 2017) to mental health and suicide (Casale et al., 2019; Kondrat et al., 2018). Through these many studies, a common theme arises—more social support provided can offer stigma reduction.

Birtel et al. (2017) analyzed the specific types of stigma and social support. Perceived stigma was found to be associated with lower self-esteem and higher depression, whereas higher perceived social support was shown with higher self-esteem and better rest. Birtel et al. suggest that substance abuse users need to have access to more-perceived social support to have less-damaging impacts on their self-esteem. As with "spoiled identity," Birtel's study supports the earlier findings that stigma can negatively impact one's personal identity and create negative health outcomes. Through these studies and many others, there is an apparent need for more social support and less stigma. The relationship between social support and stigma will be analyzed in chapter 9. Research question five described the possible differences for current and past recipients based on the different types of stigma (different types of stigma: total stigma, generalized SNAP enrollment disclosure concern stigma, past consequences from disclosing SNAP enrollment stigma, and anticipated consequences from disclosing SNAP enrollment stigma), whereas research question 5.2 is to determine if the social support received (if any) impacts enrollment on SNAP.

THEORIES TO EXPLAIN WHY CERTAIN FACTORS INFLUENCE SNAP ENROLLMENT

There may be many reasons to explain why SNAP participants experience stigma and seek social support and then disclose their enrollment to another person. To help provide some context to the many factors discussed in this chapter and the following chapters, I will briefly describe some theories of stigma: narrative theory, Relational Dialectics Theory (RDT) and the chain of discourses, and Communication Privacy Management Theory (CPM). These theories are by no means the only theories that could help explain the thought processes and dealing with stigma and social support on SNAP, but these theories provide an in-depth explanation of SNAP enrollment and relationships. I will go into further detail about the application of these theories and the factors that influence SNAP enrollment in chapter 3 and the following chapters. First, I will describe how stigma is a communicative event.

Stigma Theories

In this chapter, I introduced the importance of self-concept in understanding how people think, feel, and act on their identities. Theories of self-concept—Cooley's the "looking glass self," "salvaging the self," and Goffman's "spoiled identity"—as well as the different types of studies that have analyzed stigma helped to formalize the questions I wanted to address in this study. I will now describe the broader concept of studying stigma that was applied in my study.

Bresnahan and Zhuang (2016) suggest three classes of stigma theories: attribution theories of stigma, stigma as a power disparity, and stigma as a communicative event. Link and Phelan's (2001) attribution approach to stigma defines five stigma behaviors: labeling, negative attribution, separation, status loss, and discrimination. Though the attribution theories of stigma could be applied to my study with SNAP, the actual creation of labeling is beyond what I want to study for my dissertation but may later make an interesting study of the SNAP stigmatizer. Stigma as a power disparity focuses on the structures and social factors that create, maintain, and experience stigma. Although I will not be looking directly at power dynamics and the creation of stigma in Study 1, these social structures may be discussed in Study 2 if participants identify problems such as bureaucracy of SNAP and ease of enrollment. Lastly, stigma as a communicative event model suggests that stigma is enacted between stigmatizers and the stigmatized both verbally and nonverbally (Smith, 2007). Of all three areas of stigma research, "stigma as a communicative event" captures my primary research questions for this book, specifically how the different types of stigma and social support are communicated across social circles.

Additionally, Meisenbach's Theory of Stigma Management Communication (SMC) can help further provide how individuals deal with stigma, and "spoiled identity" while also incorporating Smith's (2007) research. According to Meisenbach, stigma communication begins with a label, mark, and so on. In this case, it would be being labeled a SNAP user. Then there is some type of stigmatizing messages whether it be physical, social, moral, and so on. After the message, the stigmatized individual determines his or her attitude toward the public belief of the mark and the applicability of the stigma to oneself. Once the individuals determine if the stigma impacts them, they can accept, avoid, evade, take responsibility, reduce offensiveness, deny, and ignore/display. These stigma communication strategies can then have outcomes that can impact health, self-esteem, achievement, and so on (Meisenbach, 2010). Though the SMC was not initially included in the analysis, several of the responses found in chapter 6 reflect the use of this theory when managing the damaging after-effects of feeling stigmatized while enrolled on SNAP, and I will provide a brief application of this theory and an indication for further study.

Narrative Theory

Narrative research is founded on the ways that humans make sense of the worlds around them, and in turn create their own individual identities and relationships (Kellas, 2008). Before discussing how narratives help define and describe the worlds around us, it is essential to describe the "differences" between storytelling and narratives. Often in research, the terms "story" and "narrative" are used interchangeably, but some researchers place distinctions on the phrases. Ochs (1997) defines a "story" as an individual event or discourse, whereas Fisher (1989) describes "narrative" as "a global frame through which to understand human behavior, interpretation, and history" (p. 242). According to Ochs (1997), a narrative is basically a broader idea than a singular story. Narrative theories are conceptualized in four primary areas of study: narrative as ontology, narrative as epistemology, narrative as individual construction, and narrative as relational process. I will briefly provide a definition of all four areas of research in narratives and then discuss the one into which this research falls.

Narrative as ontology describes how a narrative constitutes or creates our way of interacting in the world and is influenced by social factors and past history (Fisher, 1989; Bruner, 1990). Second, narrative as epistemology research focuses on how narratives can be used as a form of analysis (Orbuch, 1997). Narratives as individual construction research use narratives as a means to collect and describe stories of individuals, family interactions, and relationships. This approach to narrative research is strongly focused on the analysis of individuals' stories and the lessons garnered from them. Labov and Waletsky (1967) formed a typology for diagnosing all parts of a well-formed story including the lesson learned from that story. Lastly, narrative as a relational process moves beyond the analysis of an individual story and bases research in the interaction of narratives between the individual and the specific person in the relationship. In other words, the focus is on how audience members negotiate the story through multiple shared versions of the same story (Mandelbaum, 1987). In terms of the current study with analyzing narratives of stigma and social support, narrative as individual construction is the most salient.

Narrative as individual construction can be studied through a narrative structure approach, thematic content, or inquiry on narrative. The narrative structure approach as defined by Kellas (2008) "assigns a value to the means of constructing stories. In other words, the ability to organize a narrative according to socially acceptable criteria assumes importance" (p. 244). In terms of SNAP research, the idea of "socially acceptable criteria" is very important. Studies, as reported earlier, indicate that people feel ashamed for their enrollment and may experience disclosure concerns regarding their enrollment status. Furthermore, there is an area of research in narratives that provides a distinction between public and private narratives. While private narratives are similar to stories in which they are told individually and personally to others, public or master narratives are stories that "underlie, reflect, and perpetuate predominant cultural values and assumptions about how the world is constituted and how society functions" (Sharf et al., p. 40). The description of the master narrative could be seen as an element in analyzing the structure of narrative. The master narrative can be applied to SNAP research by analyzing stories to see if individuals report stigma from enrollment reflecting social attitudes. Furthermore, stories could be used to determine if participants believe that society as a whole distinguishes SNAP recipients as marked individuals as in felt normative stigma. The second form of analysis for the individual construction of narratives is thematic analysis.

Thematic analysis is analyzing the ways in which individuals have constructed their identities and relationship identity (Kellas, 2008). Though less applicable to the current study, thematic analysis could be used to determine themes that arise across several participants in terms of stigma, particularly perceived stigma and internalized stigma that can impact one's personal self-esteem and "looking glass self."

Lastly, the inquiry of narrative as individual construction is the most relevant for the qualitative portion of my methods and provides a method of analysis for the interviews. Inquiry of narrative "investigates the links between story structure and content and the functions these stories serve for individuals and relationships" (Kellas, 2008, p. 5). Basically, inquiry of narrative combines elements of analyzing the structure of narratives and looking for themes. Furthermore, Harter et al. (2005) define a concept called "intertextuality" which refers to how narrative meanings influence each other in ways that may not have been understood or interpreted before. Thus, the method of inquiry analysis can include how narratives were misunderstood or interpreted differently from the expected; for example, how individuals on SNAP may perceive messages of stigma directed toward them, when this may not be the case, or interpreting narratives from family and friends that may lead to more-perceived stigma. Overall, the inquiry of analysis of narratives could be used as a method of narrative analysis to determine how individuals communicate about the stigma experienced on SNAP, and their disclosure concerns may impact how they talk about these experiences with loved ones and receive social support. While there are several theories that analyze elements of narratives, one effective complex theory is RDT, specifically the chain of discourses defined by Baxter and Braithwaite (2008).

RDT and the Chain of Discourses

RDT originally formed by Leslie Baxter and Barbara Montgomery describes how communication patterns between partners are the result of opposing dialectical tensions. The overall goal of RDT is to "show how particular meanings are socially constructed and sustained through everyday communicative activities. . . . The goal of RDT is not generalizability, but rather understanding particular, studied communication" (Baxter & Braithwaite, 2008, p. 349). Further research in RDT by Baxter and Braithwaite broadened RDT to include what they describe as the "chain of discourses" applying what Bakhtin (1986) called the "chain of communion" (p. 93). Furthermore, they suggest "to do justice to the integrity of the concept of discourses, researchers will need to embed utterances in a richer 'chain of communion'" (Baxter & Braithwaite, 2008, p. 362). This "chain" occurs over three levels of discourses (a chain of discourses): history of discussion, broader cultural discourses, and anticipated response talk. History of discussion relates to how often and what past discussions have been made about a topic, specifically, how the past conversations impact and shape the future interactions. Next, the broader cultural discourse moves beyond the individual discussions to how society-at-large impacts messages. Lastly, anticipated response talk refers to how others anticipate; "Responses include those of generalized other (society in general) providing parties with a moral anchor by which to assess the appropriateness of their utterances in the present" (Baxter & Braithwaite, 2008, p. 362). In other words, participants plan on a response based on their own personal experiences with relationships as well as interactions with others in society. Now that I have described the three primary elements of the chain of discourse, I will apply each of them to the current study.

First, the past history of discourse could be applied to how individuals enrolled have communicated about their SNAP enrollment in the past. If a person and family members have talked negatively about SNAP enrollment in the past, the person may be less likely to discuss SNAP enrollment in the future. Because of the stigma that is being experienced, the person may want to talk about his or her experiences but may be unable to discuss feelings with someone because of fears or repercussions.

Next, cultural discourses could strongly influence how likely participants are to discuss stigma from enrollment. Cultural discourse can include how others in society view SNAP participants and if SNAP participants feel that others view them negatively because of their enrollment (perceived stigma, felt normative stigma, and possibly vicarious stigma). A broader example of cultural discourses can be seen in research in higher education and stigma, where the layers of shock and shame and expectations of having a higher degree and expecting higher pay lead to stigma from enrollment. These examples highlight how the chain of discourses in RDT can impact one's own identity. Thus, RDT and discourses can be applied to Goffman's (1963) work with spoiled identity in the following quote:

> The codes that are presented to the stigmatized individual, whether explicitly or implicitly, tend to certain standard matters. A desirable pattern of revealing and concealing is suggested. . . .Other standard matters are: formulae for dealing with ticklish situations, the support he should give his own (the marked individuals), the type of fraternization with normal that should be maintained, the kinds of prejudice that he should blink at and the kinds he should openly attack . . . the facing up to his own differences that he should engage in. (p. 109)

Goffman is describing the delicate process necessary in a marked individual to manage discourses that are not only intrapersonal but within one's in-group as well as the out-group. Goffman is suggesting that every individual who is stigmatized in some way organizes discourses across groups to encourage an understanding of how to deal with the stigma. With the statement "the kinds of prejudice," Goffman is also suggesting the importance of managing identity to protect the face.

Lastly, anticipated responses talk is interconnected with cultural discourses and history of discourse; if participants feel they will experience stigma from sharing their SNAP status, they may be less likely to disclose to those individuals again or may anticipate a negative response based on their past experiences with individuals and societies as a whole. When I had a stigmatizing experience at Walmart, I anticipated further stigmatizing encounters and decided to no longer use the store for groceries.

Narrative theories' analyses through the narrative structure approach, thematic content, and inquiry on narrative will provide the larger framework for analyzing the interview results from the second part of the dissertation, while, chain of discourse in RDT could be a useful tool to further narrow down the analysis of narratives by looking at the impacts of stigma and social support on SNAP and the impact of society and personal relationships.

CPM

The CPM by Sandra Petronio describes how we control our private information through a privacy management system. CPM has three main parts: privacy ownership, privacy control, and privacy turbulence. According to Petronio (2013), there are two axioms that predict how people consider their information private and how they regulate that information:

> Axiom 1 predicts that people believe they are the sole owners of their private information, and they trust they have the right to protect their information or grant access. Axiom 2 predicts when these "original owners" grant other access to private information they become "authorized co-owners" and are perceived by the original owner to have fiduciary responsibilities of that information. (p. 9)

For example, SNAP recipients may be hesitant to share their enrollment because the enrollment is considered to be stigmatizing to them, thus they may consider if they should share it at all because they own that information. Next, privacy control is the main engine of CPM; Petronio (2013) provides axiom 3 and axiom 4:

> As CPM axiom 3 predicts, because individuals believe they own rights to their private information, they also justifiably feel that they should be the ones controlling their private information. . . . CPM axiom 4 predicts that the way people control the flow of private information is through the development and use of privacy rules. These rules are derived from decision criteria such as motivations, cultural values, and situational needs. (pp. 9–10)

While there are other axioms for privacy control, these two relate to the current study.

A SNAP recipient may feel the need to control disclosing the SNAP enrollment because it is a deeply personal enrollment relating to being in poverty, a stigmatizing event. However, the individual may feel comfortable enough to share their enrollment with others, but this will follow privacy rules. These rules may be influenced by the person's situation in SNAP, the larger cultural view of SNAP (is there a larger societal stigma, racial background), and situational needs. For example, an individual may have had a negative experience at Walmart involving verbal judgment and may feel the need to share this information with someone whom they know can be trusted so that they can feel better about the situation. The situation in turn is influencing those privacy rules, but what would happen if the individual shares that information, and the person reacts in a way differently than expected; this is privacy turbulence. Petronio (2013) provides axiom 8, "Privacy regulation is often unpredictable and can range from disruptions in privacy management system to complete breakdowns" (p. 9). For example, a SNAP recipient may share enrollment with a family member and assume the person will act in one way, but when the family member does not, this may cause privacy turbulence because now the recipient has shared private information with someone who does not agree with that information. Regardless Petronio's CPM theory can provide useful insight into the disclosure of SNAP enrollment to others and the decisions to avoid discussion of SNAP.

The theories discussed—social ecological theory, the "looking glass self," "salvaging the self," Goffman's "spoiled identity," stigma, RDT and the chain of discourses, and CPM—should provide a framework to interpret and ground the results from the statistics portion of the study as well as the interview results. Chapter 3 will bring together the theories and actual statistics and interview data to broadly describe how everything fits together before going into further detail in the following chapters.

Chapter 3

Bringing Everything Together
Theory Application

In this chapter, I will discuss how I used theory to describe the results found in chapter four. To analyze how stigma and social support impact enrollment on SNAP, an explanatory sequential-mixed-methods (Creswell & Creswell, 2018) designed study was performed first with a survey to determine what stigma variables impacted SNAP enrollment; using these results, interviews were completed in to analyze how received stigma is discussed using social support. Results from the survey included 388 responses from individuals who were currently or previously enrolled on SNAP and their experiences with stigmatizing events. After the surveys were completed, 19 interviews discussing experiences on SNAP, both positive and negative were performed. Individuals from both parts of the study come from diverse backgrounds, including individuals who are immigrants, migrants, a variety of racial and ethnic backgrounds, larger households, different generations of family members being enrolled in SNAP, and higher educational attainment. Their responses are rich and complex with information about stigma and social support and are better described by applying Bronfenbrenner's social ecological systems theory, the many stigma theories discussed in chapter 2, narrative theory, RDT (the chain of discourse), and CPM. Some of the quoted interview responses may be repeated in chapters 4, 5, 6, and 7. This chapter will provide an overall view of the results from both the statistical portion and the interviews, as a generalized whole as applied to the theories discussed in chapter 2. I will go more in depth in the following chapters.

BRONFENBRENNER'S SOCIAL ECOLOGICAL SYSTEMS THEORY

As a reminder, the social ecological systems theory (chapter 2) was suggested as a method to organize the many factors that impact behaviors, and in turn are used to help develop programs by including the social environment. The Social Ecological System Theory was used to help organize the breadth of variables being analyzed in the current study. The ecological model arranges the different variables into five levels: the microsystem (individual factors affected by the immediate physical and social environment), mesosystem (interaction between systems and the environment), ecosystem (broader social, political, and economic conditions), macrosystem (larger general beliefs and attitudes shared by members of society), and the chronosystem (life events that impact individuals over the life span) (Bronfenbrenner, 1979). The results from both parts of the study can be applied to all levels of the social ecological system theory.

Microsystem factors such as migrant status, immigrant status, generation of SNAP, members of one's personal household, and the specific level of educational attainment were all significant factors that influenced the likelihood to be currently enrolled. In the interview portion, I discussed how individuals who had multiples of these microsystem factors reported more of a stigmatizing experience while being or currently enrolled than others who had fewer of those factors. The mesosystem factors can be more clearly seen in part 2 findings in which individuals discussed interactions with their friends and families providing or not providing useful support. Furthermore, individuals in the interviews also discussed how family members and friends provided judgment in their close social circles. The mesofactors in the interviews indicate how important communication about SNAP enrollment can be. For example, individuals cannot receive social support if they do not disclose to others, but if they fear a negative reaction from that person or they feel too stigmatized to do so, they will not have the positive effects that support had for some individuals. The communication with the mesofactors appears to be one of the stronger elements that impacts SNAP enrollment, because the individuals who did have positive social support systems in families and friends were more likely to not have feelings of failure, avoiding disclosure, and judgment. Next, the ecosystem factors are more generalized. To be enrolled on SNAP, one has to be 130% below the poverty line, and participants from both parts of the study were currently enrolled on SNAP, meaning they are living in poverty as defined by policy makers in the United States at this time. Furthermore, the theme of political ideology was found in three different interviews without being prompted, suggesting that the political environment does impact the view of SNAP as a whole, especially while one is enrolled. Furthermore, individuals in the interview process also reported that they see negative posts about SNAP on social media platforms, specifically Facebook; though they did not specify whom, it could be assumed that these individuals are in their social circles and not complete strangers since they befriended them on the platform. Individuals from both parts of the study reported macrosystem factors that influence their enrollment. In the surveys, one of the significant factors that loaded under total stigma was if a participant felt that society as a whole looked down negatively at SNAP participants. The societal stigma question was the only felt normative variable that was not dropped during the factor analysis, suggesting that individuals feel there is an overarching negative view of SNAP recipients. In the interviews, individuals reported the welfare abuse theme with six participants fearing being perceived as a welfare abuser by society, and eight participants reporting seeing someone else participate in abuse fraud and had a negative opinion about those individuals. Lastly, in the interviews several individuals discussed experiences that have shaped their lives after SNAP and still remember the event vividly as a chronosystem factor. While it was unclear in the surveys if individuals had lasting negative experiences because of their SNAP enrollment, the results indicated differences in reported stigma for current and past recipients. In the interviews, participants relayed stories of negative experiences on SNAP from several years ago, for one participant as much as 10 years. For example, participant 8's response referring back to when she was younger

> I can remember when I was younger and a foster kid and a teen mom, and the foster dad that I had, and I needed to get groceries, so I asked him to take to me to the store, and he was very hesitant to do so. So I asked him if we take the SNAP card and a list of groceries and go yourself if you would rather do that. He was like "absolutely not, I will not be seen with that card." It was obvious that he was ashamed to be using something like that. (Personal communication, July 10, 2020)

Similarly, participant 2 has been off SNAP for many years, and he discussed how he still feels embarrassed from enrollment,

> It was a little bit embarrassing, they would look at what you were buying. We were not like those other families out there that are buying steaks, fish, fancy foods, lobster with their food stamps. We were always aware of the looks that we would get when we would pull out the food stamps. (Personal communication, July 18, 2020)

These responses indicate that experiences on SNAP can be chronosystem factors that can impact individuals over time. This is especially salient because nine participants noted that SNAP is a temporary state, including participant 2, but he can still recall this event many years later. Overall, the social ecological system theory provides a useful framework to be able to organize the many variables that I have included in my analysis and helps provide a picture of how a multitude of factors can influence one individual with SNAP enrollment.

STIGMA THEORIES

Three theories of stigma were discussed in the literature review in chapter 2—Cooley's "looking glass self," Goffman's "spoiled identity," and Higgins's "self-discrepancy theory"—and stigma as a communicative event in chapter 3. All of the stigma theories can be applied to both the survey data and the interviews. In the surveys, anticipated consequences from disclosing SNAP enrollment stigma is a variable that formed based on the factor analysis. The questions included anticipated consequences from disclosing SNAP enrollment related to how anticipating consequences from disclosing their SNAP enrollment can impact how they view their own identity. Furthermore, all of the stigma variables significantly impacted enrollment, meaning that individuals who were currently enrolled reported a higher level of stigma from enrollment than those no longer enrolled. While results from the surveys do show support for the negative impacts of SNAP enrollment and negative identity, the interview provides examples that can be applied to each theory.

As a reminder, Goffman (1963) first conceptualized stigmas as a feeling of shame associated when a person feels he or she does not meet another's standard of behavior. Goffman's "spoiled identity" is when a discrepancy exists between an individual's "virtual" and actual identity leading to a "spoiled" social identity. Cooley's "looking glass self" is a reflection of how we think others view us. Higgins's self-discrepancy theory added to Cooley's work the idea that a discrepancy between one's ideal self and the ought self leads to low self-esteem. Lastly, Meisenbach's Theory of Stigma Management Communication (SMC, 2010) provides a framework to determine how people deal with that stigma. All of these theories are present in the themes found in the interview data. Individuals reported feelings of embarrassment, failure, fear of being perceived as a welfare abuser, avoiding disclosure, and fear of being perceived as lazy. Though I did not measure self-esteem directly, participants' responses reflect feelings of lower self-esteem when having to rely on these benefits and match some of the questions asked in the anticipated consequences from disclosing SNAP enrollment questions in the survey data. For example, participant 8 shares that she hid her enrollment from friends and significant others:

Definitely hid it from people that I work with so I don't know why because chances are, if they were working with me, they were on food stamps too. Now friends, when I was receiving benefits then I was a little bit of a party girl and so that was something that you did not want to talk about. Definitely not something that you wanted to talk about with them, anything related to domestic life. (in reference to if she was afraid any friends would judge here) No, that I feared it chances are they were on it too. When I was single and on food stamps, I did not want guys that I dated to know that I was on food stamps. . . . For myself it was a prideful thing, I wanted to maintain a certain image. I did not want something like that tarnishing my image, and destroying what little bit that I did have. (Personal communication, July 10, 2020)

Participant 8 is describing how her SNAP enrollment was at odds with her ideal self, and she feared that by disclosing this enrollment, she would "spoil" her identity and what little bit that she did have while she was poor. She is using the "avoiding—hide/deny stigma attribute" coping method described in SMC. She was concerned that if she did disclose her enrollment, people would view her differently, and thus her identity would be compromised. Participant 8's choice to not disclose her enrollment helped her protect her own image of her self-worth based on her assumptions about how others would react if they knew her about her SNAP enrollment, but this is not the case for all of the participants. For participant 19, not disclosing her enrollment did not help the inner feelings of shame and identity crisis:

First event in Vermont the social workers are exceptional awesome. I never experienced any shame or stigma from any of the social workers at all; I never experienced any overt stigma or shame in the stores that I was using the benefits in. But the overarching societal shame and the internal dialogue about needing some financial assistance equating with failure. For the internal dialogue here, I am being a highly educated person and needing food stamps was constant. (Personal communication, August 28, 2020)

Participant 19 is describing how that even without feelings of judgment from others about her enrollment, she felt that there was a broader cultural shame (macrosystem) for being enrolled on SNAP causing her ideal self to be at war with her ought self and leading to feelings of failure associated with a "spoiled identity." Participant 19 describes her "spoiled identity" clearly when she says that because she is a highly educated person, she thinks that she should not have to be enrolled on SNAP to feed her family. Initially, she describes that she is "denying" that any physical stigma occurred to her but then describes how she is "accepting" that she does feel the overall societal shame from being enrolled on the program (SMC). Both of these examples highlight how SNAP enrollment can lead to issues with "spoiled identity" and lower self-esteem with feelings of failure.

While the theories proposed by Cooley, Goffman, and Higgins deal more with intrapersonal stigma, these stigmas are socially constructed through interactions with one's social circles and society as a whole. Thus, these examples can also be applied to Smith's (2007) three classes of stigma theories—stigma and attribution, stigma as a power disparity, and stigma as a communicative event. Link and Phelan (2001) defined the attribution approach to stigma as labeling, negative attribution, separation, status loss, and discrimination. Participants in both parts discussed stigma and judgment while enrolled. Themes such as judgment and welfare abuse both relate to how some individuals receive verbal and nonverbal discrimination while they are enrolled, especially if individuals also have intersectionality of race, immigrant status, and migrant status. Furthermore, participants also report labeling as being a "welfare abuser" or "judging food choices" even if they purchase slightly more expensive items in a grocery store. The second class of stigma theories "stigma as a power disparity," though not as present as the attribution approach, can be seen in some responses to part 2. For example, participant 13 describes how the welfare system in general is built in such a way as to keep people in poverty:

> How do you shame people because they had nice cars and clothes? The welfare system was designed to keep you in bondage to it, not to get off it. It's not all about race, but still, it was so to hit the black community to keep them in need. You know they need, they were not allowed to make money and bad areas. I will put you in poverty but where do you go? The welfare system is built to continue multigenerational poverty. (Personal communication, July 27, 2020)

Participant 13 is describing how she believes that welfare and people in positions of power who shape the welfare system do it in such a way that people stay enrolled and cannot get off the programs. Participant 13 and nine others described similar incidents in which they had or knew others who had to make the decision to take another job or not and fear losing their SNAP assistance (the cutoff sub-theme under SNAP satisfaction/dissatisfaction); they chose to not take the job and know that at least their kids will be fed. Some SNAP participants reported feeling that there is a power dynamic at play with funding and continued enrollment on SNAP.

The last class of stigma theory is "stigma as a communicative event." As discussed in chapter 2, "stigma as a communicative event" is the essence of my dissertation in a whole and will be discussed further. Support from the survey data and the interviews indicate that stigmas are constructed in society about SNAP before individuals enroll on SNAP, and when they do and begin experiencing shame, discrimination, and judgment from being enrolled, they seek social support. However, as shown in the interviews, not all social support received is helpful from family and friends and can lead to feelings of failure, embarrassment, and avoiding disclosure of their SNAP enrollment. In fact, two participants suggested that the program should be stricter to allow for only certain purchases so that people would not stay on as long. Their responses suggest they feel that the SNAP program in general is full of fraud and should punish individuals on the program by allowing them to purchase only "certain" foods. This was an interesting finding because a sub-theme of "judging food choices" and "satisfaction/dissatisfaction of SNAP" was found for a more generalized society. These two individuals were sharing the stigma of SNAP enrollment with others, even though they had also been enrolled on SNAP, and one of them (participant 2) reported feeling embarrassed while enrolled. Regardless, some participants did talk about their stigmatizing or judgmental experiences with others and shared their experiences with SNAP. Overall, the current study can be seen as "stigma as a communicative event."

NARRATIVE THEORY (NARRATIVE AS INDIVIDUAL CONSTRUCTION)

The interview portion of the study allowed for the survey results to be applied to actual narratives of individuals currently or previously enrolled on SNAP. As discussed in chapter 2, narrative theories are conceptualized in four primary areas of study; the most salient to the current study is narrative as individual construction. Narrative as individual construction can be studied through three different lenses: narrative structure approach, thematic content, or inquiry on narrative (Kellas, 2008). For narrative structure approach, participants reported that they avoided disclosure of SNAP enrollment by not disclosing to others or not showing their EBT card in the grocery store because of judgment they had experienced whether from family, friends, or generalized others. The fear of being perceived as "one of those people" with fraudulent SNAP users was also found, suggesting that individuals construct narratives to "socially acceptable criteria" to avoid a "spoiled identity" to others in their social circles.

The fear of being perceived as welfare abusers (which will be discussed in greater detail in chapter 6) is also an example of public master narratives and how they can impact private narratives (Sharf, 2011). The SNAP participant is internalizing how others view the narrative of a SNAP participant and applying it to one's own internal narratives. Participants reported that they viewed social media posts in addition to family and friend comments about the negativity of being a SNAP participant and the likelihood that they are committing fraud as well, indicating that the master narrative about SNAP participants is often not seen in a positive light and can impact recipients' private narratives about their own enrollment, and thus impact disclosure. Participants reported avoiding disclosure to others, or to no one at all, indicating that their SNAP enrollment was a private narrative they felt did not need to be shared to others, specifically because of the master narrative. The master narrative of SNAP enrollment is that the program is a welfare assistance program, meaning one has to be in poverty to apply, and some fraud is committed while people are enrolled; thus, individuals are concerned how they will be viewed by society because of their enrollment. Included in this master narrative is also the political ideology component of support for SNAP as seen in three participants' responses to the theme, suggesting there may be a political factor that also influences opinion of the program, but this will need to be researched in a further study.

The second lens to analyze narrative as an individual construction of thematic analysis was the method performed to analyze the data from the interview, in which 14 themes with individual sub-themes were found. Thematic analysis allowed for the narrowing down of 19 different interviews averaging from as little as 15 minutes to over 2 hours, and with this large amount of data, it can be hard to determine what is the most important information. Thematic analysis allowed for the identification of important elements in the interview that were shared across several interviewees. Thematic analysis helped to determine elements that relate and support the survey results and offered new themes that had not been previously identified through prior research studies and pilot studies, allowing for more useful "chunks" of information and a deeper analysis of the day-to-day life of a current SNAP participant and the memories of past recipients.

The final lens to analyze narratives is the most applicable to the findings from the interviews—the inquiry of narrative. The inquiry of narrative focuses on possible links between the story structure and content and how these stories impact individuals and relationships. Considering 17 of 19 participants responded that they had received some type of social support, they definitely had discussed some elements of their enrollment with others. Yes, some participants did choose to not discuss their enrollment with particular others; the decision was often based on another response that violated their expectations. Harter et al. (2005) describe the concept of intertextuality as narrative meanings may not be understood and interpreted in ways that were expected. Intertextuality is apparent in individuals who reported negative support from their family members which leads to more feelings of embarrassment, reported judgment, failure, and laziness. Thus, individuals may have felt that they could share their enrollment status with others and receive a positive reaction but in turn did not receive the reaction they were expecting, resulting in disappointment, or as in participant 12's situation, a "falling out with the family." Intertextuality plays a key role in interpretation of messages received about their SNAP enrollment. Participants described, specifically with family or friends that were not supportive, how "shocked" they were that family and friends would communicate with them about their enrollment, and other participants reported being "shocked" at how they are judged because of their SNAP card in the grocery store. These responses were not expected and impacted how the SNAP participants viewed their own enrollment. Furthermore, intertextuality also relates to privacy turbulence in the CPM theory, which will be discussed further. Overall, narrative theories provided a broad lens to look at the interview results, but RDT and CPM theory will provide a more specific view of the findings from both the survey data and interviews.

RDT (THE CHAIN OF DISCOURSE)

RDT and the chain of discourse by Baxter and Braithwaite (2008) describe three levels of discourses: the history of discussion, broader cultural discourses, and anticipated response talk. The chain of discourse can easily be applied to the statistical findings and interview data. The significant stigma variables (total stigma, past consequences from disclosing SNAP enrollment, anticipated consequences from disclosing SNAP enrollment, and concern for disclosing SNAP to a specific person) from the survey can be seen in many of the examples provided in interviews. For example, participant 7 provides a response that has all three levels:

> Yes, I am enrolled but why did you assume? Why did this just happen? We discuss how ugly the LA card is all of the time when I am driving. I let my mom hold my card when we go in the store. In LA the card looks so cheap, whereas the Georgia is cute with peaches and looks like a card. I have never felt ashamed of; I pick and choose when I talk about, I do not publicize it. We go to a Southern Baptist with a primarily white older congregation; we are one of the only black families that go, and they probably assume that as black, we are on everything (welfare programs). It didn't make sense (that people would judge them and assume that they had food stamps) we had not had food stamps since my time as a sophomore and made over a little bit more, and cut us off. The only reason why we got it back was coronavirus, and my mom's hours got reduced and dad was furloughed. (Personal communication, July 23, 2020)

Participant 7 is describing how there is a history of judgment and stigma in which someone assumed that her mother was enrolled, and because of this, she does not publicize her enrollment with others. She also mentions that her Southern Baptist church is a largely white congregation who probably assumes that as a black family, they are enrolled on welfare assistance anyway (broader cultural discourses). Thus, she assumes from the prior history of discussion and the broader cultural discourses of SNAP and race that she anticipates a negative reaction if she discloses, so she chooses to not discuss her enrollment.

While participant 7 has chosen to not disclose to generalized others, participant 5 also provides an example in which he describes why he has chosen to not disclose to his mother as well as others:

> Actively, I go into a grocery store, you are in the line at Walmart, and I find myself trying my best to hide the fact that I am using the card. Always that fear, and in fact that more of a perceived completely hid it from my parents, especially my mom. I did not feel comfortable telling them with the exception from my father, because I know that I would have been verbally abused by mother. She would not have been happy to know that I was on it, so I hid that in shame because of that. She has talked about it in the past that people that are on SNAP are lazy people who aren't working for their money. That it is a shameful thing to rely on an entity other than yourself to receive food, I know she would have done that to me. Being from an Hispanic culture, a lot of Hispanics or minority that are on it or at least the stigma that they are on it. A lot of pride specifically from her side of the family as poor as they were, they never considered help from the government that wasn't earned. (Personal communication, July 6, 2020)

Participant 5 did not feel comfortable disclosing to his mother because of a history of discussion about SNAP participants being lazy (stigma). Broader cultural discourses also impacted his likelihood to disclose his enrollment. Participant 5 notes that being from a Hispanic culture influenced his disclosure to others because he did not want to be seen as needing help from the government because of his race and gender in the Latinx community. Because of the past history and the cultural discourse, he anticipated a certain response; thus, he chose to not disclose. Participant 5's response also brings up the issue of toxic masculinity that may also play a role in SNAP stigma. Though not a specific theme reported, participant 5, participant 8's husband, and some of the other male participants reported feelings of failure and shame; because I did not directly address masculinity in the study, I did not want to include it as a theme because I am not sure if these feelings of failure come because of gender specifically since cisgender females also discussed feelings of failure. More research needs to address feelings of failure and masculinity on SNAP, and more specifically in the Latinx community. Unlike participant 7 who continued to share her SNAP enrollment with friends who did not have a negative history of discourses, participant 5, after mentioning the worry of a reaction from his mother, shared that he never had told anyone else about his enrollment until he did the interview.

In addition to participants 7 and 5, participant 3 uses the chain of discourses to handle her interaction with SNAP and her sister-in-law:

> My sister-in-law is very against it, her and her husband are the only ones that have something negative to say about using it. . . . Now that we are all home from the coronavirus, she is really against any government help whatsoever. And talks every day about how it will ruin her business and she will have to pay taxes on it. We just do not talk about that to her or her family members so she doesn't have any reason to bring it up. To avoid the conversation altogether or the people that know her. (Personal communication, July 7, 2020).

Though a shorter example than the other two participants, participant 3 has a history of discussion (judgment and stigma) with her sister-in-law where the sister-in-law berates her for her enrollment on SNAP. Furthermore, though not referencing race as a cultural impact, participant 3 mentions that her sister-in-law does not support any governmental welfare assistance. Later in the interview, she describes how her sister-in-law judges the food choices that she purchases in the store and calls her a welfare abuser. The sister-in-law is making the broader cultural assumption that SNAP users are bad and are abusing the system. Because of the cultural discourses and the history of discussion about SNAP with her sister-in-law, she anticipates a negative response from her, so she does not disclose her enrollment with her sister-in-law, or sister-in-law's kids or friends to avoid the discussion.

All of these examples highlight that there is a process in which SNAP participants struggle with whom and how much information they should share with others; this is where the chain of discourses is particularly relevant. Participants use the history of discussion, broader cultural contexts, and anticipated response talk as a way to determine if they should disclose their enrollment to others. Though I have provided negative experiences as a means to describe the broader cultural discourses of SNAP enrollment, participants also reported having a positive history with individuals, and thus disclosed their enrollment to them and felt more comfortable doing so, as seen in participant 12:

> My parents were super supportive. My parents really helped for each bag of diapers I got they got one, cribs, they were so excited for the babies that they wanted to help in any way. My parents were the ones who told me to enroll, and that is when I signed up online. Emotional support was a small group of people my parents and some close friends I shared our struggles with individuals who also had

the same struggles themselves, so they understood what we were going through. I chose who I told the enrollment to. (Personal communication, August 6, 2020)

Before going into participant 12's experience in this quote, she had discussed early in the interview that her husband's family was incredibly combative with them about their SNAP enrollment (stigma), and went as far as to tell them that they should not have had the kids too early (a transitional state). She also referred to how she leaned on her parents to help her through their enrollment. Participant 12's parents had been enrolled in the past on SNAP and had a very different cultural view of SNAP than her husband's family, who were generally wealthier than her family. Her parents have had a history of providing help and encouragement to enroll on SNAP. Because of her family support of SNAP and her children, she anticipated a more positive response and disclosed to them. Importantly, the chain of discourse can also be visible in her decision to not disclose to her in-laws as well as to her parents.

Overall RDT and the chain of discourse is an excellent theory to help provide an example of how the thought process works to disclose one's SNAP enrollment. While RDT and the chain of discourse describes how the history of a relationship, the cultural components, and the anticipated response impact disclosure of SNAP enrollment, the CPM can help describe some of the cognitive functions at play before disclosing one's SNAP enrollment.

CPM

While RDT and the chain of discourses is applied to the specific relationships or broader cultural conversations and disclosure, CPM by Petronio describes the control of private information through a privacy management system. As a reminder, the three main parts are privacy ownership, privacy control, and privacy turbulence. Because of the cultural assumptions of SNAP enrollment and the statistical results, current participants experience more stigma because of their enrollment, it can be assumed that SNAP enrollment disclosure is a complex process in which many individuals have disclosure concerns for many reasons, and thus SNAP enrollment is not a topic that is discussed as freely as other topics may be. Participants are balancing the stigma of the program, the concerns to disclose, and personal relationships (as seen in the RDT) before they choose to disclose their enrollment. As sensitive information, SNAP enrollment also reveals that an individual is living in poverty and needs assistance to also feed the family, thus disclosure of SNAP is a deeply personal decision that is not taken lightly before disclosure. Before individuals disclose their SNAP enrollment, they have full ownership of that information; this information may only be immediately shared with a significant other or another close family member who may or may not have been present when enrolling on the program. Next, knowing the sensitivity of disclosing their SNAP enrollment, they have total control of disclosing their enrollment to others. If an individual who is enrolled weighs the past consequences from disclosing SNAP enrollment and decides to disclose, then he or she may be faced with two options: that one's privacy management was correct and the other individual respects enrollment or understands the situation and thus supports the recipient, or there is privacy turbulence and expectations have been violated from further judgment and stigma, and now the SNAP participant has to rebuild those privacy boundaries for that person.

CPM and privacy turbulence could be applied to several of the above examples, but I will provide some new examples. The first example from participant 13 describes how, because of family past experiences with being enrolled, she knew she could talk to her family about her enrollment, "My family would joke about us not trying to let others see us use the card. We share our experiences together" (personal communication, July 27, 2020). Participant 13 considered her ownership of the program, considered the history of enrollment and discussion with her family, and chose to disclose her enrollment to her family. Her privacy management boundaries were not in turbulence because her family reacted in a way in which she expected them to react, which is not the case for all SNAP participants. As a reminder, nine participants reported that they had unsupportive family or friends that impacted if they disclose to further individuals.

Participant 9 described how she is dealing with a divorce, and how her ex is threatening her with turning her into the welfare office for abusing fraud, while he is the person to whom she fears disclosing her SNAP enrollment the most:

> My ex just because of the threats, through all of that even when we were together, he wanted me to commit fraud; he said you know my sister she got a legal separation but they were still living together and got more benefits. He wanted us to do the same, I will not be paying stuff back or having prison time. It is one thing that your sister does that. It is not that it hasn't been discussed, the fact that he was accusing me of fraud when he had asked me to commit fraud. (Personal communication, July 21, 2020)

Participant 9 is an interesting example of privacy turbulence because at one time, she trusted her husband with disclosing their SNAP enrollment. Though she had been pressured to commit fraud by her husband, she did not have a violation of that privacy boundary, just that she would not commit fraud. However, once her husband left her for another woman, the dynamic of privacy changed and was thrown into turbulence because he started threatening her that he would turn her in. These threats are violations of the private information that they shared leading to turbulence in her private life as well as her SNAP enrollment she is using to feed her three children. She mentioned several times that she still fears she will get arrested or that she will have to pay the money back because of her ex-husband's actions; she cried during this discussion. Though a more extreme example, her act of disclosing private information to her husband led to a more stigmatizing experience with SNAP than she had previously, indicating the importance of controlling such private information such as SNAP enrollment from others that may abuse or further stigmatize the participant.

When combined with RDT and the chain of discourses, CPM is more salient. Individuals on SNAP refer to the history, cultural discourses, and anticipated response to determine if they can release some of the privacy ownership and transfer that to another person. When this does not go as planned, and they receive a negative anticipated response, individuals feel that their privacy management boundaries are vulnerable as seen in participants 9, 3, 5, and the other six individuals who reported their family or friends were not supportive and further stigmatized them to feel more judged or even a failure. The privacy turbulence can have devasting impacts to SNAP participants who are already dealing with multiple levels of stigma and disclosure concerns.

BRINGING IT ALL TOGETHER

I have applied Bronfenbrenner's social ecological systems theory, stigma theories, narrative theory, RDT and the chain of discourses, and the CPM to the survey and interview data. These many theories helped provide context to the rich complex data found in both the surveys and interviews. All of the theories interconnect with each other, specifically that SNAP enrollment is a complex communicative event.

The social ecological system theory helps indicate what level the social determinants of health impacted a person's life cycle. The model was also helpful at explaining how larger societal factors can impact one's personal life. Furthermore, the ecological systems model also provided a useful depiction of how all of the variables interact with each other and the power of intersectionality. All of these different factors are in play when an individual creates his or her own private narratives about SNAP enrollment.

The many stigma theories helped narrow down the large concept of stigma into usable bits of information. The works of Goffman, Cooley, and Higgins helped describe the consequences of internalized stigma from SNAP enrollment and how that stigma can impact one's internal identity.

The RDT or the chain of discourses delves into the family and friend relationships of SNAP enrollment and the decisions to disclose SNAP enrollment based on a history of discussion, broader cultural discussions, and the anticipated response to enrollment. The RDT helped to describe the importance of family and friend relationships with the impacts of stigma from enrollment, and the importance of social support in those relationships. Lastly, the CPM theory helped describe the internal mechanisms with which an individual decides to disclose or not disclose SNAP enrollment. Importantly, the CPM theory describes privacy turbulence which is found in several examples from the interview data.

Overall, all of the theories indicate that SNAP enrollment is a dynamic complex communicative event. The stigma as a communicative event was the lens of stigma theories that reflects the findings in the study. Individuals have internal factors that influence how they perceive stigma. SNAP recipients also have privacy management boundaries about their enrollment and choose to disclose who they want to have agency with that information. If that privacy management is breached, there is privacy turbulence leading to possible feelings of failure and further judgment. The privacy management is closely related to the chain of discourses present in relationships. If a SNAP recipient feels that there is a positive history of disclosure, the individual may anticipate a positive reaction if he or she tells of enrollment to another. The participant then decides whether or not to give that person access to the information. The decision to disclose enrollment is influenced by the ecological factors, privacy management, and the relational dialectics all set in the broader cultural climate and master narratives about SNAP enrollment. The decision to disclose SNAP enrollment is not taken lightly, nor is it a straightforward process because of the many factors that may encourage that disclosure such as stigma from enrollment and access to social support.

Now that I have broadly described the results from my study, and the relevant theories, in the next chapter I will briefly provide the methodological approach and results found that support the different types of stigma being present for participants who are enrolled in SNAP.

Chapter 4

Summary of Study Findings

To help provide more context from the broader discussion of theories and results from the study, this chapter will briefly describe some of the details from both the survey collection and the interviews. Further details and information from the methodological approach taken can be found in appendix B, and the survey itself in appendix G.

SURVEY FINDINGS

I recruited a total sample size of 388 participants using Amazon's Mechanical Turk engine, LSU's research participation system, and Louisiana SNAP recipients. To be considered for the study, all participants had to be a past or current member of the SNAP program. The 388 participants included a diverse sample of individuals that included 294 participants who were currently enrolled on the program for an average of 2.22 years, African American, Hispanic, Asian, Native American or Pacific Islanders, varying educational attainment, first, second, and third generation immigrants, migrant and temporary workers, varying household sizes, first, second, and third generation of SNAP recipients, and disaster SNAP recipients. For more details about the demographics of my sample, please refer to the appendix C. Overall, the sample I have collected represents a more unique and diverse sample than I have received in previous pilot studies. This diversity can inform a discussion about intersectionality and stigma across different groups who are enrolled in SNAP. Now that I have described the demographic makeup of the sample for study 1, I will briefly describe the statistical methods used.

First, a factor analysis was used to determine which of the Herek et al. stigma scale, the DISC-12, and the Wright et al. disclosure concerns scale variables may interact with each other because these variables were first used in HIV/AIDS stigma studies rather than SNAP participants. Many of the survey questions from these scales cross loaded. After conducting the factor analysis, five specific independent stigma variables loaded together: these include total stigma (Herek et al. scale), past consequences from disclosing SNAP enrollment (DISC-12), anticipated consequences from disclosure concern, generalized SNAP enrollment disclosure concern, and concern for disclosing SNAP enrollment to a specific person (for a more detailed picture of the factor analysis please refer to appendix A).

The total stigma variable is the combination of all the different types of stigma defined by Herek et al.; thus, examples of total stigma and SNAP enrollment could include being called names, physically being mistreated by customers in a store, being criticized for enrollment, hearing stories about being called names, general societal shame from enrollment, and so on.

Past consequences from disclosing SNAP enrollment stigma refer to the fact that at some point in the past, the SNAP participant has disclosed SNAP enrollment to family and friends and had an adverse experience directly linked to that disclosure. The adverse experience can include no longer communicating with family and friends or communicating less with them.

Similarly, though distinctly different from past consequences for disclosure, anticipated consequences from disclosing SNAP enrollment stigma refers to the internal fears and worries that an adverse reaction will occur if the participant discloses enrollment to others. For example, the fear of anticipated consequences from disclosure could include the feelings of needing to hide enrollment from others, fearing a negative reaction from people that they work with, or fearing a negative reaction from friends from disclosure. The anticipated consequences disclosure relates to the mental processes within one's own identity which are occurring that discourage someone from disclosing SNAP enrollment.

Generalized SNAP enrollment disclosure concern refers to more generalized fears of disclosing one's SNAP enrollment. Generalized SNAP disclosure concern describes how careful people are to disclose their SNAP status, that disclosing is risky, and the need to keep enrollment a secret. Generalized disclosure is different from anticipated and past consequences stigma because generalized does not refer to any specific event or possible event but the general mechanics of keeping their SNAP enrollment quiet.

Lastly, concern for disclosing SNAP enrollment to a specific person stigma applies to the idea that SNAP participants may be less likely to disclose to a certain person because of past experiences with that person (not necessarily about SNAP participation), and because of those experiences, they choose to not disclose as private information about SNAP to this person. While concern for disclosing SNAP enrollment to a specific person stigma is not associated with a tangible person such as a mother, father, sister, friend, and so on, the variable represents a "face" for whom the SNAP participant has disclosure concerns.

Descriptive Statistics

After completing the principal component factor analysis, I performed a cross tabulation with the Cramer's V as a measure of association for the nominal or categorical level data. Of all the categorical level demographic independent variables (IV), the highest associated with current enrollment was migrant status.

Next, a pairwise correlation was run to determine what "continuous" variables were significant with individuals who were currently enrolled as part of the exploratory nature of this dissertation. True continuous variables such as age, length of time enrolled, and members of the household are included in the analysis. Furthermore, for the sake of this research, continuous variables will include questions that use a Likert scale, such as the five primary independent stigma variables: total stigma, past consequences from disclosing SNAP enrollment, anticipated consequences from disclosing SNAP enrollment, generalized SNAP enrollment disclosure concern, and concern for disclosing SNAP enrollment to a specific person. The pairwise correlation had several variables that were correlated with current enrollment and with other variables. The following variables are associated with current enrollment: total length enrolled, members of the household, total stigma, past consequences from disclosing SNAP enrollment, anticipated consequences from disclosing SNAP enrollment stigma, total generalized SNAP enrollment disclosure concern, and total SES stigma.

Of all the continuous level demographic IV, the highest associated with current enrollment was the past consequences from disclosing SNAP enrollment, followed by the number of members of the household. Furthermore, all of the main five stigma continuous IV (total stigma, past consequences from disclosing SNAP enrollment stigma, anticipated consequences from disclosing SNAP enrollment stigma, generalized SNAP enrollment disclosure concerns, and concern for disclosing SNAP enrollment to a specific person) were highly correlated with each other. Because of the high correlations present among these variables, all subsequent logistic regression models were run separately, not as one large model, to determine what IV impact current enrollment. All of the significant variables from both the pairwise correlation (continuous IV) and the dichotomous measures of association (categorical IV) were used in the following analysis. Two variables, generation SNAP and total SES stigma, were close to significance level and will also be included in further analysis.

Discussion of the Statistical Findings

All of the following research questions and hypotheses were analyzed using logistic regression because the primary dependent variable (DV)—current enrollment status—is either a "yes, the participant is currently enrolled" or "no, the participant is no longer enrolled." The coefficient should be interpreted as a one-unit change in the IV results in the specific coefficient change in the log-odds ratio that the DV is 1. Because we do not generally think in logged odds ratios, I will be generating "predict probabilities" to help with interpretation. Furthermore, I will also provide several "goodness of fit" test results to help describe the usefulness of the model. Lastly, the models indicated a problem with the standard errors in the sample, thus robust standard errors were used. In addition to pertinent statistics information, I will provide a broad discussion of the significant demographic variables from the correlation and measures of association.

Table 4.1 includes sociodemographic characteristics of the participants in the statistics portion of the study. The size of each variable sample is detailed in the note section. Participants who completed the migrant or temporary worker question had a sample size for current enrolled of 294, and 85 for no longer enrolled. A larger number of individuals reported being a migrant or temporary worker and being currently enrolled than for those not currently enrolled. Next, individuals who were currently enrolled ($n = 289$) reported either being immigrants or descending from immigrants more than individuals who were no longer enrolled ($n = 85$). The reported highest level of education was similar across participants who were currently enrolled ($n = 294$) and no longer enrolled ($n = 91$). Lastly, individuals who were no longer enrolled ($n = 89$) had a larger percentage of first-generation SNAP users than those who were currently enrolled in SNAP ($n = 289$), whereas currently enrolled had a larger percentage of individuals' parents who had also been enrolled in the past.

Now that I have described important information about the statistical analysis, I will briefly discuss the findings broadly, and more details will be discussed in the following chapters. In my study, I had four research questions and four hypotheses, of which research question 1 is to determine which of the social determinants of health—migrant status, immigrant status, race, and education—impact SNAP enrollment; of these possible factors that may impact SNAP enrollment, migrant status and immigrant status were the two significant variables (will be discussed further in chapter 9).

Next, the findings and issues for hypotheses 1–3 and research question 2 will be addressed. After conducting a factor analysis, all of the different dimensions of Herek et al. stigma variables loaded on one factor (these variables became total stigma), suggesting that in the current study individuals

Summary of Study Findings

Table 4.1 Demographic Characteristics of Participants in Survey

Variable	Currently Enrolled N	Currently Enrolled %	Not Currently Enrolled n	Not Currently Enrolled %	Full Sample n	Full Sample %
Migrant Status						
Not applicable	62	21	60	66	122	31.7
Myself	110	37	13	14	123	31.9
Parents/Guardians	68	23	8	9	76	19.7
Significant Other	10	3	6	7	16	4.16
Other	3	1	1	1	4	1.03
Myself and parents	30	10	2	2	32	8.31
Myself, parents, and significant other	8	3	1	1	9	2.34
Significant Other and other	1	0.3	0	0	1	0.26
Myself and significant other	2	0.6	0	0	2	0.52
Immigrant Status						
Not applicable	97	34	67	79	164	43.9
First	96	33	6	7	102	27.3
Second	87	30	10	12	97	25.9
Third	9	3	2	2	11	2.94
Education						
Less than high school	18	6	10	11	28	7.27
High school graduate	31	11	23	25	54	14.03
Some college	20	7	11	12	31	8.05
2-year degree	175	60	41	45	216	56.10
4-year degree	50	17	6	7	56	14.55
Generation SNAP						
First	123	43	46	52	169	44.71
Second (parents were enrolled)	123	43	30	34	153	40.48
Third (grandparents were enrolled)	43	15	12	13	55	14.81

Notes: N = 385 migrant status. N = 374 immigrant status. N = 385 education. N = 378 generation SNAP.

do not necessarily see the different types of stigma as present in their SNAP enrollment. In other words, enrollees feel an overall sense of being stigmatized while enrolled. After removing all of the variables that cross loaded on other factors, all four of enacted stigma questions remain, such as "People have criticized me for my enrollment" and "I have been mistreated by individuals in stores because of my enrollment," suggesting that physical altercations with individuals because of one's SNAP enrollment are considered very stigmatizing experiences. Enacted stigma is the only group of stigma variables in which all factors remained after all cross loading was removed. In addition to all of the enacted stigma, two internalized, two vicarious, and one felt stigma items remained (these elements can be found in the factor analysis in appendix A). Though these elements of stigma became one variable (total stigma), it is still important to consider stigma as a whole; individuals who are enrolled are experiencing and recalling stigmatizing experiences while enrolled on SNAP. Thus, the current study does not support that Herek's et al.'s different types of stigma can be applied to SNAP participants and measuring different elements of stigma.

Unlike the issues in hypotheses 1–3, the results for hypothesis 4 were more positive. I predicted that current SNAP participants would report higher total stigma than past recipients of SNAP, and the statistical results supported this and will be discussed in further detail in chapter 6 with interview themes that also found some current members of SNAP did report more salient total stigma from enrollment.

Lastly, research questions 3 and 4 had some important findings. In research question 3, I hoped to determine how the different types of stigma—generalized SNAP enrollment disclosure concerns stigma, past consequences from disclosing SNAP enrollment stigma, and anticipated consequences from disclosing SNAP enrollment stigma—are experienced for current and past recipients of SNAP. According to the statistical results, currently enrolled individuals reported higher levels of stigma from past consequences from disclosure and anticipated consequences from disclosing SNAP enrollment stigma, whereas research question 4 is to determine how generalized SNAP enrollment disclosure may differ for SNAP participants who are currently on SNAP than those who were enrolled in the past. Generalized SNAP enrollment disclosure concerns stigma was found to not be significant. Individuals were more probable to experience stigma from a specific individual than a more generalized other. The differences across the disclosure concern stigma variables will be described in greater detail in chapter 7.

After briefly describing the statistical results for total stigma, the past consequences from disclosing SNAP enrollment stigma, anticipated consequences from disclosing SNAP enrollment, and total SES stigma, I have provided a graph of all four variables and their predicted probabilities to see the strength of the variables (see figure 4.1).

While consequences of the disclosure stigma are the strongest of the stigma variables, it is important to note that even while the probability increases for individuals who are currently enrolled to be more stigmatized, the minimum amount is higher, indicating that individuals who are no longer enrolled may still remember how stigmatized they felt while enrolled or still may be afraid to disclose their enrollment to others. Furthermore, I included SES stigma in figure 4.1 to indicate how the probability has an inverse relationship when compared to the other stigma variables. Individuals who were currently enrolled on SNAP had a higher probability of reported low levels of SES stigma, but high levels of the other stigma variables compared to individuals who were not enrolled reporting high levels of SES stigma. Though an interesting find, SES stigma will not be asked in part 2 because SES stigma was used as a controlling factor.

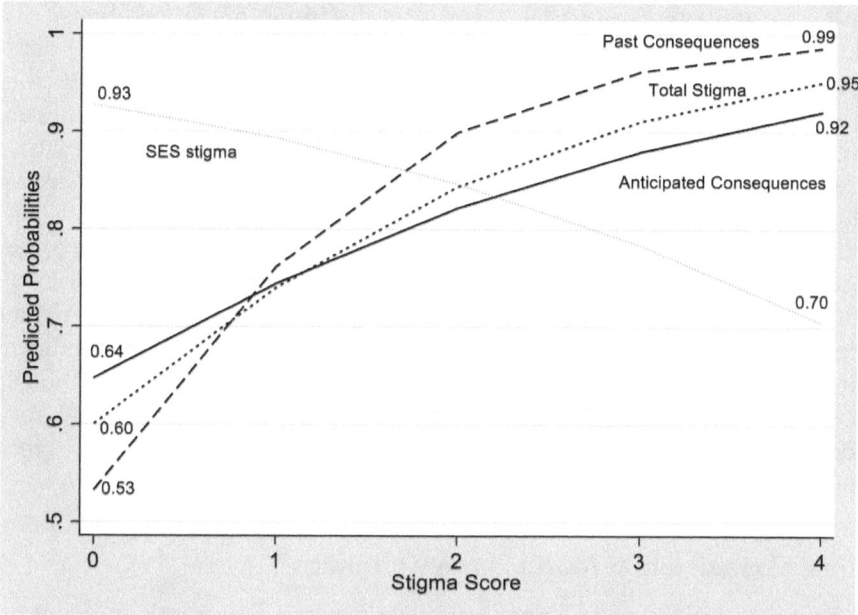

Figure 4.1 The Predicted Probabilities for Total Stigma, Past Consequences Stigma, Anticipated Consequences Stigma, and SES Stigma (IV) and Enrollment Status (DV).
Source: Created by the author.

Summary of Findings and Application to Interviews

The first part of the explanatory sequential methods design for this project yielded important results and application for the second portion of the study—the interviews. The factor analysis narrowed down the number of stigma variables from the Herek et al. scale to just one variable—total stigma. The DISC-12 variables became past consequences from disclosing SNAP enrollment stigma and anticipated consequences from disclosing SNAP enrollment. All three of the stigma variables indicate a significant difference for individuals who are currently enrolled and those no longer enrolled. In addition to the stigma elements, disclosure concern to a specific person (Wright et al. scale) was a significant factor (total disclosure was not), indicating that disclosure about SNAP is more salient when it is specifically targeted to certain individuals rather than a broad concept. These three elements were incorporated into the interview schedule to receive more details of how discussions about the different types of stigma play out in different relationship contexts. Specifically, I address any history of discourses about stigma, cultural applications, identity, or self-esteem issues brought on from anticipating a negative response from disclosure stigma, the social support received, and any past consequences from disclosing SNAP enrollment. To address intersectionality among the primary IV (total stigma, past consequences from disclosing SNAP enrollment, anticipated consequences from disclosing SNAP enrollment, and concern for disclosing SNAP enrollment to a specific person) and the demographic IV (the determinants of health), I also performed separate OLS regression models (the data is continuous for all stigma variables) for each specific significant variable—total stigma, past consequences from disclosing SNAP enrollment stigma, anticipated consequences from disclosing SNAP enrollment, and concern for disclosing SNAP enrollment to a specific person—to determine which demographic variables indicated higher stigma and higher concern for disclosing SNAP enrollment to a specific person. Note the demographic variables included in the models were determined by a pairwise correlation first, so each model may not have the exact same variables (please refer to chapters 6 and 7 for more specifics in the statistical data).

Final Consideration for the Survey Findings

I have reported these findings to provide a better framework in which to interview individuals. While questions will relate to total stigma (Herek et al. stigma scale), past consequences from disclosing SNAP enrollment stigma (DISC-12), anticipated consequences from disclosing SNAP enrollment stigma (DISC-12), and disclosure to a specific source (Wright et al. stigma scale) are necessary; it is important to determine who may feel these specific variables more saliently. Through these analyses, I have determined that larger households, migrant or temporary workers, first-generation immigrants, higher educational attainment, and multiple generations of SNAP usage are all significant factors that differ not only by enrollment but also in the amount of reported stigma and concern for disclosure.

While it is important to look at all of these variables, there are several factors I considered while interviewing. First, although minority groups did not indicate a significant finding in part 1 across any of the different types of stigma, it is important to note that while individual distinct groups such as African American, Asian American, Hispanic or Latino, Native American, and so on, are included, there was too small of sample to individually analyze these groups. Thus, there may be significant differences across groups, but this could not be determined in part 1. Furthermore, in the interview process, I recruited a diverse sample of individuals of different racial background to further analyze the differences in SNAP enrollment. Second, finding first-generation immigrants was challenging, but three were recruited in the interviews. Additionally, because of the stigma surrounding lower SES status and the stigma from SNAP itself, individuals were more hesitant to communicate, as indicated in several responses in part 2, but I conducted a snowball sample to recruit individuals from participants who were comfortable talking about their SNAP enrollment to me.

INTERVIEW FINDINGS

Procedure

Using the findings from the survey instrument, I drafted an interview schedule (see appendix D) to perform in-depth semi-structured interviews. Participants were recruited using three separate Facebook posts in which multiple individuals shared the posts. In addition to a Facebook blast, I also contacted the Office of Child Services and the LSU Graduate Association. After reaching out to these different platforms, I successfully interviewed 19 individuals (demographic information in the following pages) who were either currently or had been enrolled in the past on SNAP. Due to the nature of COVID, all individuals were interviewed using FaceTime, Zoom, or a cell phone call.

At the beginning of the interview, I asked for consent and then began recording their Zoom responses. After general demographic questions, I also told the interviewees about my own past experience with SNAP, and how I was interested to hear about their past experiences as well to determine a more rounded picture of what people's daily life enrolled as a SNAP participant is like; then the semi-structured questions began. After completion of the interviews, I reached out to another researcher who had experiences analyzing the experiences and everyday lives of individuals using interviews (Tracy, 2013; Rogers, 1961).

Demographic Data of Interviewees

Of the 19 participants, 7 were currently enrolled (37%) on SNAP, while 12 had been enrolled in the past (63%), with some being recently unenrolled (less than 1 year unenrolled). The length of time enrolled ranged from 6 months to 10 years. The average age of individuals interviewed was 34. Additionally, 5 cisgender males and 14 cisgender females were interviewed. The interviewees' racial makeup includes 12 (63%) Caucasian, 3 (16%) African American, 3 (16%) Hispanic/Latino, and 1 (5%) mixed race (Hispanic and Middle Eastern descent). Three of the 19 (16%) reported having at least one member of their household that is a temporary or a migrant worker. Similarly, three reported being a second-generation immigrant (16%). The participants reported their education levels as 3 having a high school diploma (16%), 11 with some college (58%), 4 masters or professional degrees (21%), and 1 doctorate (5%). The household size of interviewees varied from 1 dependent to more than 5 dependents; 6 of the 19 (32%) had more than 5 family members. Lastly, many participants had been enrolled on both SNAP and D-SNAP (58%, 11), and 8 had been enrolled on SNAP only.

Analysis

After transcribing all of the interviews, we began initial coding. After comparing results and making changes from earlier trials, we narrowed down to 14 themes. The 14 themes were: embarrassment, temporary enrollment, necessity or survival, race, a transitional state, avoiding discussion of SNAP enrollment, assuming failure, judging food choice, politics (conservative versus liberal), assumed laziness, social support, judgment, satisfaction/dissatisfaction with SNAP, and welfare abuse. Using these 14 themes, we coded all transcripts. To measure interrater reliability, Cohen's κ is used (for more information about the interrater reliability, please refer to the appendix E). Through the iterative process, the 14 themes can be further described by applying Bronfenbrenner's social ecological systems theory, RDT, Petronio's CPM theory, and Goffman's Theory of Self discussed in chapter 3. All responses in the following themes that mention names are pseudonyms. Please note that due to the complex intersectionality in participants, some themes are interwoven and may be present in a singular example or may be used more than once.

Themes

Table 4.2 presents the 14 themes from the codebook with example quotes, frequency, and κ score. Themes are listed from the most mentioned to the least mentioned.

Now that I have described all 14 of the specific themes found during my analysis, I will briefly provide an explanation for the research questions I analyzed for the interview questions, as in the statistical results, with more details provided in the subsequent chapters. Once again, after completing 19 interviews, 14 specific themes were found: satisfaction/dissatisfaction with SNAP in general, social support, judgment, avoiding discussion, welfare abuse, embarrassment, necessity/survival, a transitional state, hiding the card, temporary enrollment, race, judging food choices, laziness, failure, and political ideology.

As with the statistical portion of this chapter, I formulated two research questions. For research question 5.1, I was interested in determining how/if the different types of stigma (total, past consequences from disclosing

SNAP enrollment stigma, anticipated consequences from disclosing SNAP enrollment, and concern for disclosing SNAP enrollment to a specific person) found in part 1 using the survey would be described in experiences for current and past recipients and if there were any noticeable differences between the two. First, all 4 different types of stigma can be found in the 19 responses. The themes of judgment, welfare abuse, judging food choice, embarrassment, laziness, failure, and avoiding discussion of SNAP enrollment all relate to the different types of stigma. I will provide a brief explanation from these themes that matches all four different types of stigma and discuss further in chapters 6 and 7 (avoiding disclosure).

As a reminder, in part 1 findings, all four types of stigma (total, past consequences from disclosing SNAP enrollment stigma, concern for disclosing SNAP enrollment to a specific person, and anticipated consequences from disclosing SNAP enrollment) indicated a significant difference between current and past SNAP recipients. Though the relationship was weaker for anticipated consequences from disclosing SNAP enrollment and concern for disclosing SNAP enrollment to a specific person, the relationship was significant. Part 2 findings do not suggest a large difference between current and past recipients, because both mention feelings of judgment or shame from being enrolled. However, there are some interesting statements that do suggest a difference between current and past recipients, and I will go into further detail in chapters 6 and 7. For example, for total stigma, current members who had been enrolled in the past, and they were off for a period of time and now had reenrolled, reported experiencing more stigma the second time being enrolled than the first time. Next, only one participant reported having severe past consequences from disclosing SNAP enrollment to others. As in the statistical results, participants did not seem to have a preference to whom they were most concerned with disclosing their SNAP enrollment, unless there was a history of judgment. Lastly, the statistically significant findings from part 1 reflected the responses for individuals who anticipated consequences from disclosing SNAP enrollment. All of the findings for research question 5.1 will be discussed further in chapters 6 and 7.

While it is important to consider the stigmatizing experiences of an individual enrolled in SNAP and the possible ramifications, understanding how social support received from members of one's social circles impacts enrollment both negatively and positively is vital as well. Research question 5.2 was formulated to answer the question of how social support received (if any) impacts enrollment on SNAP. In general, there does not seem to be one type of social support that is more favored for individuals while they are enrolled on SNAP, but there are significant impacts for positive and negative social support, and the source of that support (family versus friends). The impacts from social support will be discussed in greater detail in chapter 8.

Table 4.2 Themes from Interviews Code Book (N = 19)

Theme	Example Quotes	Frequency, n (%)	κ
Satisfaction/ dissatisfaction with SNAP	"I think it is a great program.... I think it is a program that is very valuable for desperate situations." "But when you get down to it, it helps so many individuals and families who otherwise would struggle with feeding themselves and their families, so because of that reason, I feel like it's an important and very necessary program that I'm grateful to be able to participate in. Actually, I feel that the guidelines and requirements should be stricter in order to reduce fraud and abuse of the benefits." "I joined the military, I go to apply to food stamps. I made 36 cents too much. Mr. John, we are so sorry can I give you a dollar every month, even though we needed it and we are suffering. It is difficult for folks who are struggling, and they have to decide if they should take this job and stay on food stamps at least my family has food."	18(95)	0.63
Social Support	"YES. We would talk about my situation, married with two kids and having a hard time finding employment; it was a little bit difficult. Talking to family about and to take advantage of the programs that are out there ... Family and friends were supportive but did not give us any money or anything." "So I asked him (foster father) if we take the SNAP card and a list of groceries and go yourself if you would rather do that. He was like 'absolutely not, I will not be seen with that card.' It was obvious that he was ashamed to be using something like that."	17(89)	0.82
Avoiding discussion of SNAP enrollment	"All of my close friends except maybe one does not know I feel a need to hide it (SNAP). I have never considered it, but I have never explicitly told him that I have food stamps. I never considered why, but now that I think about, he is very upper middle class, I just do not know how he would react. I am very uncertain." "Not that I am aware of, I still have not disclosed that to anyone. Other than receiving disaster benefits from the flood of 2016." "We just do not talk about that to her or her family members so she doesn't have any reason to bring it up. To avoid the conversation altogether or the people that know her." "You can tell the ones that are ashamed because they swipe their card long before the cashier ever finishes ringing them up ... I have hurried up and swiped my card so the person behind me doesn't see you swipe the card."	16(84)	0.89

Summary of Study Findings 61

Theme	Quote	n(%)	
Judgment	"Oh yeah, I would call my mom in tears, and she would be like why are you letting these people get to you and you do not even know them. I said I don't know it is just so embarrassing to be in the line at the grocery store, but they always sigh or make some type of snide comment." I have heard them say, "She is buying shrimp, lobster, and all that expensive stuff, and she is buying all that on food stamps." "My wife's family know how to work the system; they suggested that we get on SNAP even though I did not want to, and I was ashamed. They mocked me and said I was riding the disability train because of my injury."	15(79)	0.93
Welfare abuse	"We were not like those other families out there that are buying steaks, fish, fancy foods, lobster with their food stamps." "I know some people use the funds to trade for things they do not supposed to, and I know others that are doing the wrong thing. I get why she thinks it is the wrong idea; that is not what we do. We literally just feed our children, we do not buy crap to get through the month. She says so you are affording steaks?" "My ex just because of the threats, through all of that even when we were together, he wanted me to commit fraud. He said, 'you know my sister, she got a legal separation but they were still living together and got more benefits.' He wanted us to do the same, I will not be paying stuff back or having prison time."	14(74)	0.89
Transitional state	"We would talk about my situation married with two kids, and having a hard time finding employment; it was a little bit difficult." "Now that we are all home from the coronavirus, she is really against any government help whatsoever."	13(68)	0.84
Embarrassment	"I knew that I needed, I did not like being on it. My wife and I had a child unexpectedly while we were still in school. I had just started my masters while she was in her bachelors." "I view myself as very pragmatic. I knew that I needed it; I could have been emotional about, but I knew that I needed to feed my family. It was a mix of shame, fear." "I pull out the EBT card and immediately my face got hot, and I had to pull out the other EBT card. At that moment what it felt like to be totally reliant on food stamps and how shameful." "It was a little bit embarrassing; they would look at what you were buying."	13(68)	0.88

(Continued)

Table 4.2 Themes from Interviews Code Book (N = 19) (Continued)

Theme	Example Quotes	Frequency, n (%)	κ
Necessity or Survival	"... it was helpful for us and made it possible for us to survive instead of starving to death." "And even though I actually did need the help, since I did not look like I needed the help, I felt looked down on for using the government." "Honestly I do not talk to a lot of my family, my mom and sister that I know, they know my situation and they know that I need it."	13(68)	0.83
Temporary enrollment	"We explained to them that it is a temporary thing, we did not plan on staying on it forever." "Friends and others, mostly how it is ok to be enrolled in it. This is a temporary thing; it is ok."	9(47)	0.75
Race	"I think there is a connotation of a black woman that has food stamps. They just do not know. You cannot just not work on and get SNAP." "Being from a Hispanic culture, a lot of Hispanics or minority that are on it or at least the stigma that they are on it." "A white lady behind me said oh look another one using the government. It is just so rude, I was totally shocked."	7(37)	0.96
Judging food choices	"Last week I wanted to buy a sub sandwich from the store, and you know that you cannot buy a hot sub with your stamps. I wanted a hot sub, and I knew that I did not want to eat it right away. In my mind I wanted to ask them to not heat it up. I was afraid to ask it ... I paid 10 in cash that I did not even like, but I could have got in my food stamps, and I would have liked. Even though she would not say it to me, in my mind I thought she was going to think it." "Yes. Or even on Facebook!! They should not be allowed to buy steak and they should not be allowed to buy shrimp, should only buy beans and rice, you know things like that!"	6(32)	0.87
Laziness	"I have family members on both sides, while they supported me at the time knew of my situation, but still would make comments about social programs and how they thought it was, I guess, used for lazy people." "She has talked about it in the past that people that are on SNAP are lazy people who aren't working for their money."	6(32)	0.94

Failure	"No one wants to admit that they need any help. I felt a lot of I am a failure. I can't provide. I can't stand on my feet." "But the overarching societal shame, and the internal dialogue about needing some financial assistance equating with failure."	4(21)	0.83
Political ideology	"One of those typical offensive conservative lines, #comebackwhenyoucontribute, as if paying taxes is the only way to contribute, as if you do not pay taxes when you are on SNAP, even though we did." "I am a remote worker; my people I work with are not in the same state and one is very liberal, so he probably would support it."	3(16)	0.91

In this chapter, I provided a brief and broad overview of the results and methodologies used in the study. This chapter offers a more concise view of the results that will be discussed further in the following chapters and a general understanding of the breadth of results found in this large study. Before I can discuss the complex findings about the stigma and social support on SNAP, in chapter 5, I will provide some broader SNAP themes that help describe how stigma can form.

Chapter 5

General Views of SNAP Themes

Chapters 3 and 4 provided a broader view of the study as a whole and provided a brief explanation of findings; this chapter begins a deeper inspection of the results. In this chapter, I will discuss how broader themes found in the interview data help explain some of the elements of stigma that can occur from SNAP enrollment. Before understanding the negative impacts of stigma and how those feelings of shame and embarrassment could then impact the disclosure of SNAP enrollment, it is important to delve into participants' views of the SNAP program as a whole—the satisfaction versus dissatisfaction of SNAP, enrollment in the program as a necessity and survival, enrollment as a transitional state, and that enrollment in SNAP is temporary. All of the following responses came from the interview data.

SATISFACTION/DISSATISFACTION WITH SNAP

The satisfaction/dissatisfaction with SNAP theme relates to the participants' views of SNAP as a whole. Out of 19 participants, all but one responded with an opinion about the state of the SNAP program, which is to be expected because the last question in the interview was "How do you feel about the SNAP program in general?" The theme had several sub-themes: the program is valuable, the program does not cover enough (meaning the program needs more options, such as covering baby food, formula, and diapers), rigid cutoff rules (the amount needed to stay enrolled is too rigid), and other issues. Seven of 19 participants reported multiple sub-themes.

SNAP Is Valuable

An example of SNAP is valuable can be found in the response of a 33-year-old white cisgender female with two dependents (participant 18) who said, "The SNAP program really saved our skin those two years" (personal communication, July 18, 2020) or in a 36-year-old Hispanic cisgender male with three dependents (participant 5) response,

> I think it is a great program. I think with any program that provides financial assistance, I am sure that there are plenty of people that fit whatever stigma who abuse the system having kids to be on the system. I think it is a program that is very valuable for desperate situations. (Personal communication, July 6, 2020).

In addition to participant 18, participant 1 (38-year-old African American cisgender female) also discusses her support of SNAP with some discussion of other issues with the program:

> I am def a supporter. I def see how it is a benefit for those who are low income. I wish there was more resources for those families who do struggle with feeding their families. I feel that education is crucial too. I feel that is missing when people receive benefits. Those resources when they no longer in need of that assistance. I am def an advocate for it. Definitely a person who educates people on the program, I told an individual last week who was having trouble getting access to food, that based on your income that you could qualify in SNAP. Something that they could think about. (Personal communication, July 10, 2020)

Participant 1 is describing how she feels that the program is very helpful for individuals who are low income and that more education should be available to low-income individuals to encourage enrollment in a program that would help them. She also describes that she has shared information about the program to others.

Participant 5, a cisgender Hispanic male with two dependents, found that while the program may be hard to get on, the advantages were also present:

> It is difficult to get on it but when you get on it but the support you receive is pretty good. The follow up interviews were not a bad experience the people were very professional. When my time was up, when I finally got a job to support the family, I got off of it there was no feeling of being forced out the door but you are own your now. They went out of their way to help the money I had coming in was the national guard and money from school, the income did not count as income were counted as seasonal and not permanent. We were initially denied and we filed a claim and when they researched it, they found that we

did actual qualify. They actually could have said no you do not qualify but it to help us and get us the money needed. (Personal communication, July 6, 2020)

These examples highlight the opinion that overall the program is positive and can be a very helpful tool for individuals who are living in poverty, but for the other sub-themes, this positive sentiment is not reflected.

Rigid Cutoff Rules

In the SNAP program to be enrolled, an individual must have an annual income that falls below the 130% of the poverty line; if income goes above 130% at any time, the individual is unenrolled in the program. At this time, there is not a program to help individuals after they no longer qualify. This rigid cutoff point was found in several responses such as in that of participant 4, a 21-year-old white cisgender female with no dependents:

> They make it very hard who is not to use the government to use the government. If I make $1300.01, you cannot apply for it. Literally, that is $10 an hour, and that is before taxes are taken out. I think it is stupid. I went to apply for it with the $1100 after taxes, but because I made $1300 before, I could not get it. And I was bad off and hungry and needed it but could not. (Personal communication, July 8, 2020)

Participant 13, a 39-year-old African American cisgender female with seven dependents, described an instance when she was visiting family in Louisiana:

> When I was back in LA visiting family, we wanted some crawfish, and one of my old friends told me that she had quit her job because they were going to take her food stamps away. Are you kidding that you quit your job because you fear losing your food stamps? But then I thought I understand her. The system is set up to let her think that way. Because she was working a job, and she was not making that much money on the job, but she was making enough to cut her food stamps. But without the food stamps, I would not be able to feed my children if I keep the kids. Because I am penalized for working so she quit her job so she could have food stamps. (Personal communication, July 27, 2020)

Participant 3, a cisgender Caucasian female with seven dependents, describes her frustration with the allotments given on the program:

> I think it is a great program especially if it used the way that it is supposed to used. A lot of people would not survive without it and a lot of people do not

get enough for what they need. A dad and her daughter only get 86 month what does that buy milk? Well it is hard to live off of that, it is not more difficult to buy and cook for 7 than it does for 2. Harder for smaller families. (Personal communication, July 7, 2020)

Participant 12, a cisgender Caucasian female with two dependents, also voices her frustration with the rigid guidelines:

You know it sucks already. It's not like you want to be using it or that it is a fun time. You are struggling this is why you qualify for it. They are very strict on the income. When Jeff started making $30,000, we were kicked off and you know we were ok with that but we still struggled. It would have been better if they would have provided something small. So when someone says it needs to be more stringent, I am like just get out of here, they are already pretty strict. (Personal communication, July 10, 2020)

These examples highlight the desperation of needing to still have the aid from SNAP to provide food for their children but faced with the decision that if they earn more money, they will no longer be enrolled. Additionally, there also seems to be a fear that if I do make more than what is allowed, I will lose what I have, and then struggle to feed my family with what I am making. In total, 10 participants noted that the SNAP program as a whole places undue restrictions on when a person has to unenroll and forces individuals to make hard decisions of finding employment.

Other

For the other sub-theme of satisfaction/dissatisfaction of SNAP, participants may have reported differences among states and enrollment such as participant 3, a cisgender female from New Mexico, who explained, "Never any question of how it works or what we need. It has been easy here" (personal communication, July 7, 2020), and in a 20-year-old African American student's response,

"I told my mom and she said I should have applied as a freshman. I had to apply twice but my residency is in Georgia but I work in Louisiana, where do I apply. They said Louisiana and while I am at school, my permanent address in Louisiana. They first denied me because of the address, this is a minefield. (Personal communication, July 10, 2020)

In addition to differences across states, one participant, a cisgender male who had been enrolled many years prior, reported on how time has impacted enrollment, "It was easier to enroll back then than it is now. If you met the criteria you qualified, this is what you get. They were giving it to everyone back then."

Participant 15, a 52-year-old cisgender female also describes some frustrations with SNAP and age,

> It was good as people in need, however it does not make sense to me that even if you are $50 over, they will kick you off it. I think that it needs an allowance period before getting off. It doesn't make sense to me that it hurts people who are in need that are so close to the cutoff amount. (Personal communication, August 3, 2020)

Some more examples that fit the other category for satisfaction/dissatisfaction with SNAP may include how helpful some agencies are at helping push people through the enrollment process (participant 8), the uncleanliness of the SNAP office (participant 8), dependents being too old to receive benefits, but still live in the household (participant 11), the welfare system being designed to keep you in bondage (participant 13), and so on. For example, participant 8 describes in greater detail that she feels that the process of enrolling in SNAP can be improved if people are more helpful:

> The most effective help was when an agency walked me through it. It is frustrating there is a lot of ins and outs for things to come together. Sometimes agencies will help push the paper work through. The help is greatly appreciated. You walk into this huge gigantic faceless building, it is sterile you know, you walk in and it is dirty and it smells and there is 100 of people and you can smell the people. It is not a judgment thing, it is just intimidating you are shoved all of these papers, the secretary does not want to talk to you. You are stuck in line for 3 "fricken" hours and your kids are crying and hungry. It's horrible, if you go to the drop box there is a chance they will not get it, you have to be do it there to do it. They are so unforgiving about missing that phone call. It is terrifying too because they will cancel it while you are relying on it. (Personal communication, August 6, 2020)

Participant 8 is describing how she feels if there was someone there to help that the process would go smoother and would be less daunting. Specifically, she also notes that the building was not clean and was loud, which added to her feelings of shame for being enrolled. Participant 8's response does reflect what other responses were included; participant 13 also describes how she feels the SNAP program is formulated in such a way to keep people enrolled:

> The welfare system was designed to keep you in bondage to it, not to get it off it. It's not all about race, but still it was so to hit the black community to keep them

in need. You know they need, they were not allowed to make money and bad areas. I will put you in poverty but where do you go. The welfare system is built to continue multigenerational poverty. (Personal communication, July 27, 2020)

She is expressing how she feels the program is flawed by adversely encouraging the African American community to be enrolled, thus indicating her dissatisfaction with the program. Now that I have provided several examples of satisfaction/dissatisfaction with SNAP, I will include combinations of both satisfaction and dissatisfaction together.

Combinations

Some participants reported combinations of the sub-themes, such as participant 2, who is a 50-year-old white cisgender male with four dependents:

> I think it is a good program for those that need it. The issue I have with the program overall is that is does not limit you on what you buy such as blue crab that I saw on a YouTube video where a woman used food stamps to purchase the crabs. I was on food stamps when I was a young minister, $400 a week as a youth pastor. I joined the military; I go to apply to food stamps I made 36 cents too much. "Mr. Tom, we are so sorry. Can I give you a dollar every month?" even though we needed it and we are suffering. It is difficult for folks who are struggling, and they have to decide if they should take this job and stay on food stamps at least my family has food. If you do go over the monthly limit, then have a grace period in which you are on a 3-month period. (Personal communication, July 18, 2020)

Participant 2 is discussing how valuable SNAP is with saying that it is a good program for those that are in need, whereas he is also discussing the issues with a rigid cut-off line for individuals who have to make the choice to stay on SNAP and not to take a new job, or take a new job and lose SNAP, but still need the benefits. Lastly, his example is an "other" as well because he is discussing how SNAP also needs stricter guidelines to control what is purchased, which is in contrast to what others have said about lessening the restrictions to be able to buy things like baby food.

Another example of a combination of the sub-themes would be participant 13, an African American cisgender woman with seven dependents:

> They take the money that you have in the bank, and they add it to your income. What they got off your pay stub. This does not make sense because if I get paid and I get a check for $600 and I have to hold that because my rent is $1200, this cannot be used for food. Thus, the money gets counted twice, even though you

cannot spend it, so people lie that there is not any money in the bank account so that they can get SNAP because we cannot use that money. If someone gives you $300 to help towards your rent one month, and you tell them, that will be taken out of your monthly snap benefit. That is not your income. It's like the rules are not applicable to who needs it. I have several friends who left their jobs to be on the program because they wanted to do more but their hands were tied. (Personal communication, July 27, 2020)

Participant 13 is discussing cut-off issues again with the discussion about friends that she knows who had to choose between the program and a job, whereas the discussion about declared income would be in the "other" subtheme because she is discussing the issues with qualifying for SNAP in the first place.

As the most mentioned theme by participants, in general SNAP participants do see the program as valuable, but with some challenges. Regardless of the dissatisfied feelings of the programs, participants also reported that enrollment is a necessity for survival.

NECESSITY OR SURVIVAL

The necessity or survival theme is how participants view the program as a necessity or a need to help them survive a difficult time in their lives. The theme was coded for the presence of either the words "necessity" or "survive" or statements such as "to feed my children." Of the 19 participants, 13 reported the need or survival component of being enrolled in SNAP. Participant 6, a Hispanic, cisgender male with four dependents, describes how a period in his life led to a need for SNAP, "Relieved. Because without that benefit, I would have a difficult time being able to provide enough groceries to feed my family. We've faced some serious financial hardships the past 5 years" (personal communication, July 9, 2020).

Participant 12 also describes a need for SNAP after having a child, "Right after the kids were born, I got on both SNAP and WIC; we could not afford the food and diapers that came with twins" (personal communication, August 6, 2020). Participant 8 also voices a need for the program while taking care of a child,

> It was with people who needed help figuring out what to do. Cause at one point, we were struggling pretty bad using all of the system, so when I find other people single mom struggling, I feel like I am capable to explain how to make their situation a little bit better. (Personal communication, July 10, 2020)

Participant 13, a African American cisgender female, shares that when she needs the program, she wishes she was not as stigmatized:

> I have always hated the food stamps program personally, yet I work in this country and pay into the system, so when I need the program that I can use it. I do not care if people think that I need it because I am lazy. I do not like the program because I do not want to have to need it. I am not against the program, but I do not want to be on it. (Personal communication, July 27, 2020).

Clearly, all of these participants are describing how they used SNAP benefits when they were at their most vulnerable and could not provide for their loved ones, but might still feel shame in the process of needing the program. Many of these examples included a need for the program because of a transitional period in their lives.

A TRANSITIONAL STATE

As was expected, 13 of the 19 participants reported some type of event that suggested that SNAP was a "stepping stone" to a better point in life. In other words, enrollment on SNAP was a transitional state or point in one's life. An example of a transitional state would be that of participant 7, a 20-year-old African American cisgender female, "They all understand, we are all struggling college students, but I do hear it in passing" (personal communication, July 10, 2020). Participant 7 is in a transitional state because she is currently a college student who is focusing on her studies and not working several jobs, whereas participant 9, a 33-year-old Hispanic cisgender female, is having relationship struggles, "Most of the time people will not say anything, but the moment you pull out the card people seeing it. Ok, so they do not know my story, that my husband took off with another woman" (personal communication, July 21, 2020). Participant 9 is discussing the aftereffects of feeling stigmatized after her husband left her with three children and with no source of income; thus, she needed to enroll on SNAP. A final example of SNAP enrollment as a transitional state can be seen in participant 11 (a 52-year-old white cisgender male), "I always had made a lot of money, but I had a back injury, and I had to quit my job" (personal communication, July 23, 2020). All of these participants and others reported that SNAP enrollment was because of a specific event that was occurring in their lives at the time that made it necessary to enroll in SNAP, and implying that their situation has improved or will improve in the future so that they will no longer need SNAP as a financial support.

Though similar to transitional state, participants also reported that SNAP enrollment is only temporary. Fewer participants also reported that SNAP was temporary than a transitional state.

TEMPORARY ENROLLMENT

Unlike transitional state, where a specific incident is described for the reasoning why the individual needs to enroll, such as unplanned pregnancy, job loss, or an injury, temporary enrollment individuals specifically say that their enrollment is temporary or imply that enrollment on SNAP is not long-term. Nine participants suggested that SNAP was only a temporary enrollment; five interviewees specifically use the term "temporary" to describe their enrollment, as in participant 5's response:

> I talked about the stigma differently with my significant other than with my dad. We talked specifics with significant other, and talked about the funds and arguments about the use of this. A personal level. With my father, I always spoke of it as means to an end, a process. It is temporary; there is a lot of great things about it; I can get this, I can get that. (Personal communication, July 6, 2020)

Similarly, participant 12 describes her enrollment as

> we explained to them that it is a temporary thing; we did not plan on staying on it forever. Jeff was finishing up medical school and we get residency money so it was only for a two-year period in which we needed help with food money. (Personal communication, August 6, 2020)

Participant 18, a cisgender Middle Eastern descent male described specifically that enrollment is temporary, and that one must work hard to make sure that it is only temporary:

> This is a temporary thing it is ok. Now because there is a lot of churches who gives out food, look thank God I have a little bit of money so that I do not go and take other people's food. I was not going to take advantage of the situation and hurt someone else's chance. Thank God I have a little bit, and that is ok to get some if you need it. That is what I tell them about SNAP it is ok to need to get on it. You know it is a like a Sh*** apartment, you know it is okay to stay in one for the time, but work towards something better. Someday I will get out of this, I will work harder and get better (Personal communication, August 20, 2020)

Comparatively, participant 2 does not directly state that his enrollment was temporary, but his word choices suggest that he feels as a whole that enrollment on SNAP should be short-term, "I thought it was a necessary program that was struggling. I do not believe that we should be on it for years and years. We should be working to get off food stamps" (personal communication, July 18, 2020). Another example of not specifically using the term "temporary" but meaning a short-term enrollment would be when participant 7 jokes with her friends in college:

> I do not see it as a source of shame, because we talk about it a lot. My food stamps are coming on the 15th, in fact mine is coming in 5 days. That is my brother's birthday, and I will go get a cake. We will talk about when do you get your funds, I got that food stamp card. We joke about it all of the time and it is more fun, they are not judging me because they are either on now or about to be on it. You will not be on it forever. (Personal communication, July 10, 2020)

While the temporary enrollment theme is distinct from the transitional state theme, they are interrelated. A transitional state may be needed to enroll on SNAP in the first place, but there is the assumption that the enrolling on SNAP is a temporary state until the situation improves, and they no longer need to be enrolled.

The four mentioned themes in this chapter—satisfaction/dissatisfaction, necessity or survival, transitional state, and temporary enrollment—are general views of SNAP as a whole, but these views also reflect an understanding that the program is a need, but that it can also come with problems, especially if an individual sees the program as temporary or transitional. In fact, some of the responses in this chapter have reflected some feelings of stigma, such as participant 13 stating how much she hates the program, but still has to be enrolled, or participant 5 that says he talked differently about the program with different members of his family. It is essential to understand the broader views of SNAP as a whole before delving into the stigma and shame associated with being enrolled, especially in terms of being dissatisfied with being enrolled, and the feeling that one is relying so much on a program that has caused him or her to think about self-identity while enrolled. Some of these feelings of dissatisfaction with the program and the necessity for survival can lead to participants reporting issues with stigma in chapter 6.

Chapter 6

Stigma and SNAP Enrollment

In chapter 4, I provided interview themes that described some general views of SNAP; some see the program as valuable but with some issues that led them to have feelings of shame and embarrassment. In chapter 2, how stigma was first conceptualized by Goffman in 1963 is explained. Stigmas are the feelings of shame that are associated when a person does not meet another person's assumption of what the appropriate person should look like. For SNAP participants, the stigma comes from being enrolled on a welfare assistance program such as SNAP, in addition to other factors that impact enrollment such as race, migrant status, and immigrant status. Initially, there were several stigma measures that were used to measure different facets of stigma that were narrowed down into total stigma, past consequences from disclosing SNAP enrollment, anticipated consequences from disclosing SNAP enrollment, generalized SNAP disclosure concern, and concern from disclosing to a specific person. Overall, this chapter will briefly provide the statistical results that support how individuals feel stigmatized when they are enrolled on SNAP, then follow with the interview themes, and conclude by tying in the statistical results and the interview data in order to examine the impact of stigma on SNAP enrollment.

OVERALL FINDINGS

In the analysis, I determined that individuals who were currently enrolled had higher overall scores of total stigma, past consequences from disclosing SNAP enrollment stigma, anticipated consequences from disclosing SNAP enrollment stigma, and concern for disclosing to a specific person. The only stigma variable that was significant was generalized disclosure concern stigma. Furthermore, there were also significant differences in individuals who were members of several different groups. For example, individuals who were an immigrant, a migrant, had larger households, and higher educational attainment all reported higher levels of stigma than individuals who were not members of those groups. Additionally, participants who also had multiple generations of family members who had been enrolled in SNAP also reported more stigma than other groups. Most pertinent is that individuals who reported being members of multiples of these groups appear to experience the most stigma while they are enrolled in SNAP. However, the statistical results for individuals who are no longer enrolled are still sometimes high, considering these individuals are not living daily enrolled on the program. The results indicate that stigma experienced while enrolled on SNAP is a dynamic process that does not impact all individuals the same. Furthermore, my findings support my past research as well as other research in the field that indicate people do feel shame and stigma from being enrolled on the program. Now I will go into greater details about specific findings in the statistical analysis.

DETERMINING THE IMPACT OF TOTAL STIGMA

The first part of my statistical analysis was to determine if current members of SNAP would experience more total stigma than individuals who were no longer enrolled; this was found to be statistically significant (hypothesis 4). Results from the hierarchical logistic regression are presented in table 6.1. The second nested model for total stigma was significant (Wald χ^2 (8) = 59.29, p = 0.000), indicating that total stigma did differ for those who are currently enrolled and past enrolled. In addition, total length, migrant status, immigrant status, generation SNAP, and members of the households all significantly differed by status of enrollment. Total SES stigma and generation SNAP were also close to significance level ($p < 0.10$) and will be included in the discussion.

To further illustrate the effect size of the significant variables, I will provide the maximum and minimum differences of generated predicted probabilities for all variables. The largest change in the predicted probability of being currently enrolled was the number of members living in the household utilizing the benefits of SNAP (predicted probabilities [0.55,0.98]) for a positive change of 0.43). Households with more members relying on the benefits were more likely to be enrolled.

The second largest change in predicted probability is total stigma (predicted probabilities [0.59, 0.95] for a change of 0.35). Individuals who were currently enrolled were more likely to be experiencing larger amounts of stigma from SNAP than those who were no longer enrolled. The predicted probabilities

Table 6.1 Hierarchical Logistic Regression Results for Total Stigma (IV) and Enrollment Status (DV)

Variable	b	OR	95% CI for b LL	95% CI for b UL	Robust SE b	Pseudo-r²
Step 1						
Constant	−1.23***	0.29	−2.01	−0.45	0.40	0.26***
Total length	0.19*	1.21	0.04	0.35	0.08	
Migrant status	0.55**	1.73	0.17	0.94	0.20	
Immigrant Status	0.64**	1.90	0.18	1.10	0.24	
Education	−0.01	0.99	−0.29	0.28	0.15	
Generation SNAP	−0.39^	0.68	−0.81	0.05	0.22	
Members of the household	0.59***	1.80	0.29	0.88	0.15	
Step 2						
Constant	−1.35	0.25	−2.27	−0.43	0.47	0.28***
Total length	0.19*	1.21	0.03	0.35	0.08	
Migrant status	0.48**	1.62	0.13	0.83	0.18	
Immigrant status	0.52**	1.67	0.06	0.97	0.23	
Education	−0.01	0.99	−0.29	0.27	0.14	
Generation SNAP	−0.52^	0.60	−0.97	−0.06	0.23	
Members of the Household	0.58***	1.79	0.27	0.90	0.16	
Total SES₁	−0.35^	0.71	−0.71	0.02	0.19	
Total Stigma₂	0.64**	1.89	0.18	1.10	0.24	
Goodness of Fit						
Cragg-Uhler/ Nagelkerke r²	0.41					
Wald's X² (df = 8)	59.29					
% Predicted Correctly	0.81					
PRE	0.29					

Note: CI = confidence interval; LL = lower limit, UL = upper limit. Pseudo r^2 = Mcfadden's. PRE = Proportion reduction in error or a null model. N = 282. ^p < 0.10, 'p < 0.05, ''p < 0.01, '''p < 0.001. ¹DISC-12 scale'; ²Herek et al. (2013) stigma scale.

indicate a higher total stigma for those enrolled than for those no longer enrolled. There is a higher probability that those who are currently enrolled will report a higher total stigma score than those no longer enrolled. Individuals currently enrolled reported a mean total stigma score of 2.20 (SD = 0.93) compared to those who were no longer enrolled (M = 1.50, SD = 0.77). While these total stigma scores seem low, a tabulation indicated that 40.3% of those who were currently enrolled reported moderate to the highest stigma score, whereas 10% of those no longer enrolled reported moderate-to-high stigma. Thus, in the current sample, individuals could be reporting high stigma or very little.

Next, individuals who had single or multiple members of the household who were a migrant or temporary worker had a higher predicted probability of being currently enrolled (predicted probabilities [0.72, 0.99] for a change of 0.27). In other words, individuals who had single or multiple members of the household who were a migrant or temporary worker had a higher predicted probability of being currently enrolled. For total length, participants who were currently enrolled had a higher probability of being enrolled longer on the program than those who were no longer enrolled (predicted probabilities [0.78, 0.99] for a change of 0.21). The last positive relationship, immigrant status, indicated that households who had an individual who was an immigrant were more probable to be enrolled on SNAP than those who were no longer enrolled (predicted probabilities [0.77, 0.94] for a change of 0.17). Both generation SNAP and total SES stigma had a negative relationship with individuals currently enrolled. Individuals who were currently enrolled had a higher probability of lower total SES stigma than individuals who were not currently enrolled (predicted probabilities [0.73, 0.92] for a negative change of 0.19). Similarly, individuals who were a first-generation SNAP user had a lower probability of being currently enrolled than individuals who had other family members enrolled in the past (predicted probabilities [0.72, 0.88] for a negative change of 0.16).

To help provide more context into how different social determinants of health could impact stigma, another model was run with total stigma. The model was significant ($F_{(7,293)} = 18.37$, $p = 0.000$), with migrant status (b = 0.09, Seb = 0.03, β = 0.15), immigrant status (b = 0.22, Seb = 0.06, β = 0.21), education (b = 0.12, Seb = 0.05, β = 0.14), generation SNAP (b = 0.12, Seb = 0.06, β = 0.20), and members of the household (b = 0.11, Seb = 0.03, β = 0.18) all having significant higher levels of stigma when compared across groups. The β scores indicate the effect size each variable has on total stigma; immigrant status appears to have the strongest effect size, with generation SNAP being slightly less.

Participants who reported as being or having at least one individual living in the household who is a temporary or migrant worker had higher total stigma levels (M = 2.23–2.56, SD = 0.97–1.13) compared to those who were not temporary or migrant workers (M = 1.44, SD = 1.09). Also, the more members of the family who were also migrant or temporary workers, the higher the reported stigma.

The next significant indicator in total stigma was immigrant status. If the participants were first-generation immigrants, they had a mean stigma score 2.57 (SD = 0.80) compared to those who were not first-, second-, or third-generation immigrant (M = 1.51, SD = 0.88).

After migrant and immigrant status, education was also a significant predictor, but not as strong a relationship as the previous two. The higher the educational attainment, participants reported having higher stigma (M = 2.22, SD = 1.01) than those who had less educational attainment (M = 1.62, SD = 0.87).

Generation SNAP is an interesting finding because in the above logistic regression with current enrollment, generation SNAP was often a negative relationship indicating that individuals were more likely to be currently enrolled if they had family members who had also been enrolled in the past. However, in the overall stigma regression, individuals with family members who had also been on SNAP reported having higher stigma (M = 2.20–2.34, SD = 0.93–0.89) than those who did not (M = 1.74, SD = 0.97).

Lastly, one of the strongest independent variables from the logistic regressions, members of the household, also is present in total stigma. Participants with more household members that rely on SNAP reported having higher stigma than individuals with small households. A household with more than six individuals had a mean total stigma score of 2.22 (SD = 0.67), whereas a single individual household had a mean total stigma score of 1.37 (SD = 0.76).

For total stigma, the results indicate that individuals who are migrant or temporary workers, immigrants or have family members who are immigrants, higher educational attainment, a multiple generation SNAP participant, and larger households all should be included in the interview process because of the possible higher levels of stigma when compared to individuals who are not. Overall, the groups that were found to be more significantly stigmatized than others were recruited for the interview data, and similar results were found from the 19 individuals who were interviewed. Now that I have briefly mentioned the statistical results that support the stigma for current individuals enrolled on SNAP and the different social determinants of health that are also more stigmatized, I will provide the interview responses that reflect the stigma experienced on a daily basis while enrolled on SNAP.

STIGMA INTERVIEW THEMES

In addition to the statistical data that found people experienced stigma from being enrolled on SNAP differently per the individuals, the interview data also supports these findings. Several themes were found in the interview data that reflect stigma on SNAP is a complex event. Themes relating to stigma experienced while enrolled include feelings of judgment, embarrassment, and failure. In addition, individuals reported being accused of or know someone who had committed welfare abuse. Lastly, participants reported accusations of being lazy or selecting poor food choices in the store. A closer analysis of the data and the participants also indicate, as in the statistical data, that participants who were immigrants, migrant workers, members of larger households, and so on, reported having higher levels of stigma from these events, especially if they were members of more than one of these factors. All of these examples paint a complex image into the lives of individuals who are enrolled in SNAP and the impacts the program has on their daily lives beyond the purchasing of food.

Judgment

Judgment is the fourth largest theme with 16 participants responding they have felt like they were judged for being enrolled in SNAP. The judgment theme relates the closest to the three main stigma variables found in part 1. During the iterative process, four sub-themes were found: perceived judgment, actual verbal judgment, actual nonverbal judgment, and combination of the three. Perceived judgment relates to the feeling of being judged for being enrolled on SNAP such as the feeling of stigma from the society at large from being enrolled on SNAP. Actual verbal judgment is when an individual actually communicates verbally some insult about being enrolled in SNAP to a SNAP recipient. Actual nonverbal judgment would be the intentional eyes rolling, scoffing, or staring while judging a SNAP recipient. Lastly, there are several participants who reported combinations of the three sub-themes of judgment in their interviews. First, I will provide examples of perceived judgment, then actual verbal, actual nonverbal, and combinations of judgment.

Perceived

Of all 16 participants, 13 participants had perceived some judgment from being enrolled. The perceived theme relates to the feelings of judgment or stigma from being enrolled in general, not judgment tied to a specific event. Participant 1, an African American cisgender female, provides a good example of perceived judgment from the society at large for individuals enrolled on SNAP,

> I can tell that we live in a society that stigmatizes individuals who do enroll in food stamps and that is horrible. A large part of it is the lack of education is missing. We basically put a band-aid on a wound that is bleeding instead of

getting to the root of what is the issue and how we can help people. (Personal communication, July 10, 2020)

Participant 1 is not directly referring to herself, because she mentions that she did not feel judged or stigmatized herself while she was enrolled in SNAP because she did not disclose to others that she was enrolled, but she is acknowledging that people do feel stigmatized because of their enrollment. Participant 1 is describing how she chose to "isolate herself" (SMC) of her stigma, by choosing to not disclose at all to others to help protect her self-esteem, but she acknowledges that others after displaying their stigma, may feel more stigmatized than before.

Another example of perceived judgment can be found in this response of participant 2, a Caucasian cisgender male, to the name of the program: "In my day I was enrolled on food stamps, now it is SNAP. I think there is a stigma to the name itself" (personal communication, July 18, 2020). Participant 2 is referring to the name of "food stamps" or "SNAP" itself as being stigmatizing. Participant 2 also did not say that he had experienced any stigma from being enrolled, but he acknowledges that people do feel stigmatized and judged while they are enrolled. Participant 2 is suggesting that he was accepting of the stigma that he was experiencing; he also used humor as a means to ease his discomfort while he was describing his history with the program, even though he said he did not experience any stigma.

Lastly, participant 9 also emphasizes the stigma in general she felt from being enrolled on SNAP,

> I need it so I take advantage of it; if you do not need, do not take advantage of it. Unfortunately, the stigma is definitely still there, you will still be frowned upon. It doesn't matter what you look like. If people would just have more compassion for each other or physically attacking you or anything like that. (Personal communication, July 21, 2020)

Unlike participants 1 and 2, participant 9 discussed several times in her interview that she felt stigmatized for her enrollment, but her example here is acknowledging the stigma at large for being enrolled on SNAP, no specific examples. Perceived stigma reflects the assumption that individuals face stigma from just being enrolled, not through any direct statements made to them, but just from a generalized view of SNAP by the society at large. Next, some examples of actual verbal judgment are provided.

Actual Verbal

Similar to perceived judgment, 13 participants responded with an example of actual verbal judgment directed specifically to them as a person and their

82   *Chapter 6*

SNAP enrollment. For example, participant 13, an African American cisgender female, said,

> To be honest, they see a young black woman with kids, they automatically assume/think you are food stamps. They automatically categorize, they automatically think you are lazy. I have a lot of people in the grocery store I was in at the time, and the lady made a comment the food choice that I was making, "It's good to see that at least you are buying healthy food." I mentioned something about my husband, and she said "Oh, you are married. I would never have assumed that you were married because you were not wearing your ring." She had never seen my hand to even know that I was not married. She had automatically assumed that I had all these babies by different men to get food stamps. (Personal communication, July 27, 2020)

Participant 13 is describing an actual encounter that occurred in the grocery store regarding her SNAP enrollment; the other individual specifically commented on what was in her grocery cart. She is also describing the importance of her race and those assumptions and statements that she has had to endure in the grocery store.

Similar to participant 13, participant 9 also has an example of an actual encounter in the grocery store in which someone was physically assaulted:

> I am sure that people have way worse experiences than me, 'cause I know it happens. I have read stories online about it. One lady was fostering some children and they did not have any clothes or anything like that. She brought them to Walmart in an attempt to pay for everything. And the guy behind her starting attacking her . . . so she was trying to buy food for the night using food stamps because it was an emergency situation that she had got into and she did not know what to do. When the guy behind her starting attacking, she just broke down. . . . These events can happen at any moment, all they have to do is look at you and assume things and it happens all of the time. (Personal communication, July 21, 2020)

Participant 12, a Caucasian cisgender female, also discusses verbal interactions in grocery stores:

> When I would get in the line at the supermarket with the kids, you would hear all of the comments about using the EBT card and the WIC vouchers. They would sigh and say there is another one; that happened one time at a Winn-Dixie in Gretna. A white lady behind me said, "Oh look, another one using the government." It is just so rude, I was totally shocked. This has happened more

than once, and at different stores too. One time it was a Walmart, Albertsons. (Personal communication, August 6, 2020).

Unlike participants 12 and 13, participant 10, a Caucasian cisgender female, mentions actual verbal judgment from friends, "Definitely with friends mentioned about applying in April, 'That must be nice, too bad the rest of us can't get it.' So that I did not continue. I cannot wrap my head around it; we are both not working" (personal communication, July 21, 2020). Participant 10 not only states that she was verbally judged from a friend because of her enrollment, but that after this event, she chose to no longer disclose her SNAP enrollment to anyone.

Lastly, participant 3, a Caucasian cisgender female, discusses a verbal encounter with her sister-in-law about the type of food she could afford with SNAP,

> I get why she thinks it is the wrong idea. That is not what we do, we literally just feed our children; we do not buy crap to get through the month. She says, "So you are affording steaks?" No, we literally just have hamburger meat and pork chops. Do you have any idea on how much we pay for groceries? (Personal communication, July 7, 2020)

She in some ways is using the "reducing offensiveness" tactic under SMC by using the "bolstering/refocusing" tactic of indicating to her sister-in-law that she is only using SNAP to provide food for her children.

All of these examples describe encounters of feeling judged from being enrolled on SNAP because of a verbal discussion. These participants provide a breadth of examples of when verbal discussions have occurred, and some share how stigmatized they feel because of their enrollment and these statements directed to them. Next, I will provide examples of nonverbal judgment.

Actual Nonverbal

Comparatively, fewer participants reported actual nonverbal judgment from others (5 out of the 16). An example of actual nonverbal can be found in participant 2, a Caucasian cisgender male. He says, "We were always aware of the looks that we would get when we would pull out the food stamps card" (personal communication, July 18, 2020). Participant 2 is specifying the looks he received when he was in the checkout counter in a grocery store.

Participant 7, an African American cisgender female, also reports eye movements in the grocery store, "But I do know that people will side eye you. Why? I feel very lucky with the friends that I have that say you do what you gotta do" (personal communication, July 10, 2020). Both participants are highlighting the looks received while in the grocery store, not direct statements of judgment as in actual verbal. More examples of actual nonverbal judgment can be found in combinations of judgment.

Combinations

In total, eight participants mentioned some combination of perceived, actual verbal, and actual nonverbal judgment. Participant 5, a Hispanic cisgender male, provides an example of perceived and actual verbal judgment from a family member and society at large:

> You look at people while you are on it, at least the perception of, you hear people snickering, or any noise, and think "Yep, they saw the card and they see that I am on it they think that I am using the system." I hid it from my parents, especially my mom. She has talked about it in the past that people on SNAP are lazy people who aren't working for their money. That it is a shameful thing to rely on an entity other than yourself to receive food. I know she would have done that to me. So I hid that in shame because of that. (Personal communication, July 6, 2020)

He is describing perceived judgment when he discusses how he looked at people for their responses when he was enrolled, while the actual verbal judgment came from his mother about SNAP participants being lazy and how it is a shameful thing to rely on the government for food. Based on these past experiences, he chose to isolate himself and not discuss the stigma with others (SMC).

Participant 8, a Caucasian cisgender female, describes an encounter in a grocery store in which she experiences both perceived and actual nonverbal judgment:

> We all got ready and went to the grocery store; I felt fine, and I knew the moment was coming to pull out that card. I was really excited to maybe get food that we had not been able to get because of the Covid virus. When we get to the cashier, $300 was gone so I pull out the EBT card and immediately my face got hot, and I had to pull out the other EBT card. At that moment what it felt like to be totally reliant on food stamps and how shameful to think that if I do not have money for this, I will have to put stuff back which is also embarrassing. Now, I know that the cashier does not care, the little old lady with the Coach bag behind you is staring at you, and the bagger is staring at you, and immediately I thought, "Man, I do not miss being on food stamps." (Personal communication, July 10, 2020)

Participant 8 is describing perceived judgment when she is describing how she became so embarrassed about what others would think if she needed to put items back and being reliant on SNAP, whereas the actual nonverbal judgment comes from the looks from the bagger and the little old lady.

Participant 9 provides an example that includes all types of judgment—perceived, actual verbal, and actual nonverbal. Participant 9, a Hispanic cisgender female, describes multiple incidences:

> Most of the time people will not say anything, but the moment you pull out the card people seeing it. Nothing is ever said to me, but you can see the sideway glances or the cashier that is kind of looking down on it. Oh, you are a white woman with kids, you should not be in need of governmental assistance. It's mostly the looks, no one has really ever said anything about it. But just the looks that they give you, you can tell what they are thinking. There is an incident in which my mom was in the post office, and there was this young girl and her mom that graduated around the same time that I did. She was with my young son who was a toddler at the time. I was already pregnant with my second. They just turned around and said, "You know that she is on WIC and food stamps. I can't believe that she is pregnant again without being married," and all of that other stuff. And my mom this definitely does happen, and they were not white, they were African-American. It happens all of the time. (Personal communication, July 21, 2020).

When participant 9 highlights the feelings about pulling out the card and about being looked down on for being a white woman and needing assistance, she is describing feelings of perceived judgment, whereas when she specifically mentions the cashier looking at her differently in the store, that is nonverbal judgment. The verbal encounter with her mom and a past classmate about her enrollment on SNAP and WIC is an example of actual verbal judgment.

One final example that highlights the next theme of welfare abuse and actual nonverbal judgment can be found in participant 2's response, "It was a little bit embarrassing they would look at what you were buying. We were not like those other families out there that are buying steaks, fish, fancy foods, lobster with their food stamps" (personal communication, July 18, 2020). He is highlighting how he is not "one of those people" who abuses the system, but at the same time, he feels judged for being enrolled and being viewed as "one of those people." Participant 2's statement includes the next theme of welfare abuse, or the assumption that SNAP participants are welfare abusers because they are enrolled on a welfare assistance program.

Welfare Abuse

Welfare abuse was mentioned by 15 of the 19 participants and refers to four sub-themes: the fear of being perceived as an abuser, being asked to commit fraud, seeing others abuse SNAP, and other examples. According to the USDA,

> USDA works to make sure that only those families who are actually eligible for the program participate, and that the correct amount of benefits is provided to them. Over the past decade, USDA has made major strides to improve the accuracy of SNAP's eligibility determination and benefit payment system. . . . Stronger Rules. USDA published a final rule in August 2012 that requires states to cross check against the Social Security Master Death File, Social Security's Prisoner Verification System, and FNS's Electronic Disqualified Recipient System prior to certifying individuals for the program, to ensure that no ineligible people receive benefits. ("What is FNS Doing to Fight SNAP Fraud?", 2019)

In addition to stronger rules, the USDA notes when people fear that too many people abuse SNAP, the public has a lower opinion of SNAP as a whole:

> While it occurs relatively infrequently, USDA recognizes that program fraud undermines public confidence in government and the program. This jeopardizes the ability of SNAP to serve over 20 million struggling families who currently need it the most. USDA works through our state partners to investigate recipient fraud and hold bad actors accountable. Recipients who purposely commit fraud to get benefits are subject to disqualification. Fraud investigations yield results for taxpayers. In fiscal year 2011, states completed nearly 798,000 fraud investigations, resulting in over 46,000 disqualified individuals and collection of over $72 million in fraud claims. ("What is FNS Doing to Fight SNAP Fraud?", 2019)

To provide a different perspective for welfare fraud, Aussenberg (2018) found in a Congressional report that for every 10,000 households participating in SNAP, only four would be investigated and charged with SNAP fraud because of the rigorous process to be enrolled on the program, but U.S. society still believes that SNAP abuse is prevalent. These beliefs can be found in the following examples.

Fear of Being Perceived As an Abuser

The fear of being perceived as an abuser sub-theme relates to how individuals worry about being seen as a possible abuser of SNAP benefits or the welfare system as a whole. Six participants out of the 19 reported a fear of being perceived as an abuser. For example, participant 2, when he discusses how he is not one of those people, feels the need to justify that he is not abusing the program.

Participant 4, a cisgender Caucasian female, also fears being perceived as an abuser of the program. She says,

> Oh yea, no one has ever said anything directly, but I drive a Lexus. I would go with my card, and no one really knows, but I paid $10,000 out of pocket and it is used. I would go and pay and feel that everyone looks at me, especially the public. And even though I actually did need the help, since I did not look like I needed the help, I felt looked down on for using the government, even though it is here for us to use. (Personal communication, July 8, 2020)

Participant 4 is worried that if someone sees the type of car that she is driving (A Lexus is generally seen as a luxury car) and knows that she is on food stamps, the person would likely accuse of her using the system for extra money to pay for food, when she can afford an expensive car.

Participant 9, a Caucasian cisgender female, also voices the need and the discouragement from being perceived as a welfare abuser:

> It makes you feel discouraged. I have only ever used it when I needed, I never have tried to fool the system or anything like that. I literally use it if I need it. I take what I need. 100% honest with them all of the time, when I do not need it, I call and cut it immediately so I do not have to pay back all kinds of money. Again, I never play the system, but right now with three dependents and me by myself, it is just something that I need. (Personal communication, July 21, 2020)

Participant 9 is an example of a fear of being perceived as a welfare abuser because she continually reiterates that she only uses it when she needs it, but that she feels bad for having to need it.

While the examples for the fear of being perceived as an abuser relate more to the perceived stigma defined under judgment, some participants reported being asked to commit fraud and saw others commit fraud themselves.

Being Asked to Commit Fraud

The theme of being asked to commit fraud is straightforward; if an individual reported ever having been asked to commit fraud, the person was coded in this sub-theme. Expectedly, only three participants responded that they had been asked to commit fraud while enrolled in SNAP, but I found their responses to be very important since fraud is considered to not be as prevalent as expected. Participants 7 and 13, both African American cisgender females, shared a story in which they were both asked to commit fraud over the telephone. Participant 13 states,

> This one lady in my social circles, she calls me on a different number so I did not know who it was a first. She told me and we were talking and I was thinking, "She must need something." She asked me, "Do you have any food stamps for sale? Didn't I buy them from you a year ago?" I said no, are you sure? I said it had to be someone else. Now granted that this was just a few weeks ago and I was getting it, I did not tell her this specifically. I told her besides even if I did, I would not sell them to you. I want it all for myself! LOL! The fact that she had the audacity to just come to me to assume. She assumes that I have seven kids I was on food stamps. Then she was like, "Oh save my number this is my new number." I thought Oh sure I am definitely going to save your number now that you insulted me. Then she asked me "Do you know of anyone that is selling?" I have a mutual girlfriend that I had to call to tell her about the story. How does someone who I have never had the discussion about food stamps have the balls to call someone else based on assumption and ask can you sell? (Personal communication, July 27, 2020).

The act of SNAP fraud mentioned in the response of participant 13 is the act of selling one's food stamps for cash or other monetary gain. Participant 9, a Caucasian cisgender woman, mentions an instance in which her ex-husband was asking her to commit fraud,

> He wanted us to do the same, I will not be paying stuff back or having prison time. It is one thing that your sister does that. It is not that it hasn't been discussed, the fact that he was accusing me of fraud when he had asked me to commit fraud. (Personal communication, July 21, 2020)

Participant 9 is describing an occurrence in which her ex-husband confronted her when they were together and attempted to persuade her to commit fraud because they knew of someone else who was doing it; after they separated, he then is accusing her of fraud, which will be discussed in a following sub-theme. Though not as prevalent as the other sub-themes, being asked to commit fraud provides profound insight into the cultural components of the stigma surrounding SNAP participants.

Seeing Others Abuse SNAP

Eight interviews describe instances in which recipients have seen others abuse SNAP. Abusing SNAP can consist of buying or selling SNAP for money and using SNAP funds to buy drugs, and so on. Participant 6, a Hispanic cisgender male, describes more generalized that people do commit fraud and should be punished for it:

> As with any type of government assistance, it's not perfect, some take advantage of it and abuse it. . . . People complain about the paperwork, deadlines, and requirements but really it's a small price to pay for what it provides. Actually, I feel that the guidelines and requirements should be stricter in order to reduce fraud and abuse of the benefits. It's a benefit, not a right or entitlement, so I'm willing to do whatever is required to stay enrolled and because it's a benefit, I depend on it to feed my family. (Personal communication, July 9, 2020)

While participant 6 is more generalized about abuse, participant 9 describes an instance in which an individual who was enrolled in a local co-op committed fraud:

> I am now recalling a parent actually telling me about how she was able to stay on SNAP benefits though she exceeded the financial guidelines. She and her siblings would work a second job for most of the year; at about the 6-week mark (before SNAP reconsideration was about to occur), they would quit their second job to make it look like they hadn't been making that extra money. They would get another temporary second job until it was time to re-apply for food stamps. I don't have an opinion about this method, but I do recall that it was important for parents who brought their children to the daycare to get ANY BENEFIT THEY COULD, and they would stop at nothing to get it. Mostly, I remember that with this particular family, they were very outspoken about it and seemed not to be ashamed at all. (Personal communication, July 10, 2020)

Similarly, participant 11, a Caucasian cisgender male, also provides an example of specific people who have abused the system:

> I definitely still feel that fraud is happening today. I knew a gentleman who was getting food stamps and he had won a settlement (large) and still drew benefits. Jane was collecting $600+ a month for mom, her, and child and she drew disability and her mom drew state retirement. I also had coworkers who were drawing a similar paycheck to mine, and they would sell food stamps for fifty cents on the dollar in order to purchase alcohol. I do not misuse that I would have to pay it back, and I don't want to go to prison over something as minimal as food stamp fraud. (Personal communication, July 23, 2020)

Lastly, participant 13 describes an instance in which she knows that a friend is committing SNAP fraud, but she is doing it to help her family:

> Unfortunately, people sell their SNAP, but they do it because there is a need. If you are selling your stamps to keep the lights so the food does not go bad, it's kind of a catch 22. I am not so hard to say she doesn't deserve the food stamps. Not as many people sell their food stamps sell for drugs, I am not stupid that people can sell it for that. But people are selling it to take care of their kids. (Personal communication, July 27, 2020)

Other

For the other sub-theme, any mentions of welfare abuse that did not fit the other sub-themes are considered. Five participants responded with "other" information about welfare abuse. For example, participant 19, a Caucasian cisgender female, critiques people's viewpoints about fraud on SNAP,

> and as far as fraud, that amount is so small and negligible when compared to corporate fraud. And the misplaced angry people who get angry for using their 0.005% of their tax dollars versus where they should be really upset where their taxes dollars are going to. (Personal communication, August 28, 2020)

Participant 5, also mentions tax and fraud:

> I think it is a great program. I think with any program that provides financial assistance, I am sure that there are plenty of people that fit whatever stigma who abuse the system having kids to be on the system. I think it is a program that is very valuable for desperate situation. It is not meant to be a permanent thing, people take advantage of it, but people will take advantage of everything. It's what our taxes are supposed to be paid for; it is supposed to help people that are in need. (Personal communication, July 6, 2020)

Participant 7, a cisgender African American female, describes how black women are stigmatized as welfare abusers, "Probably I just do not want them looking at me. I think there is a connotation of a black woman that has food stamps. They just do not know. You cannot just not work on and get SNAP" (personal communication, July 10, 2020).

Overall, while the total amount of SNAP fraud may be lower than is reported by the USDA, individuals do know of some that committed fraud on the SNAP program, or they feel more stigmatized because they do not want to be seen as a person that abuses the program. The abuse of SNAP does seem to indicate that people feel some disdain toward individuals that do, or at least that they do not want to be identified as a SNAP abuser. The perceived abuse of SNAP adds another level of stigma for individuals who are enrolled on SNAP. The next theme relating to stigma, judging food choices, has been briefly suggested in some of the prior examples of stigma.

Judging Food Choice

In the actual verbal theme, participant 13 mentions that she was told "It's good to see that at least you are buying healthy food." Her description is the assumption by the general population that individuals who are on SNAP all purchase either junk food (cokes, chips, candy, etc.) or superexpensive food like lobsters. Of the 19 participants, 6 participants mentioned having someone else judge their personal food choices. Participant 16 (a Caucasian cisgender female) describes how when she worked at Walmart, she saw several individuals comment about the contents of a person's cart:

> I have heard people, especially when I was a cashier at Walmart, individuals who had buggies full of groceries with things that they could not buy. And you would hear them say, "Well, you know they are on food stamps." I have witnessed that a lot. Off-hand, I remember comments about "Well those people are on food stamps." Or even on Facebook!! "They should not be allowed to buy steak, and they should not be allowed to buy shrimp, should only buy beans and rice." You know, things like that I have seen on Facebook and have got upset over that, even though I am not currently on it. Like what? I am not supposed to feed my kid any snacks? Those items are cheaper, what do they expect us to be able to eat? Frozen pizzas and snacks are cheaper than fresh fruit and vegetables. It is ridiculous with how people view SNAP recipients. (Personal communication, August 3, 2020)

Participant 16's response accurately describes the theme of judging food choices, meaning that someone is telling another person on SNAP what they should and should not buy, and if they do buy that item, they are judged for purchasing it. She also highlights that the judgment does occur not only in the grocery store but also on social media platforms.

Participant 13's response indicates agreement with participant 16 with overhearing customers in grocery stores judge a SNAP recipient's food purchases,

> Sometimes, especially when I am in the store, I know what types of statements the cashiers make because I used to be a manager of several retail stores. I have heard them say "She is buying shrimp, lobster, and all that expensive stuff, and she is buying all that on food stamps." (personal communication, July 27, 2020)

These examples and others indicate that individuals on SNAP are also judged for the food choices, specifically shrimp, steak, lobster, frozen pizza, crabs, snacks, healthy expensive food, fish, and energy drinks. It appears from these responses that SNAP participants have a catch 22 effect with the food they purchase; if they purchase cheaper foods such as frozen pizza, they are seen as unhealthy, whereas if they spend more SNAP benefits to receive healthy foods, they are also shunned for spending too much on those foods.

These stigmatizing events that have occurred to participants, whether verbal, nonverbal, or perceived, can lead to feelings of embarrassment, perceived laziness, and even feelings of failure. Thus, after these events have occurred, participants feel a wave of emotions that impact how they see themselves as they are enrolled on SNAP.

Embarrassment

The embarrassment theme relates Goffman's theory of "Spoiled Identity." Specifically, in chapter 3, I describe how Goffman (1963) defines stigmas as the feelings of shame associated when a person feels he or she does not meet another's standard of behavior. Goffman (1963) also describes the idea of "spoiled identity" where the stigmas create a sense of personal devaluation and in turn impact how the person sees one's own individual identity. Spoiled identity can then impact how people see themselves and how others see them as well. Additionally, Charles Cooley's "looking glass self" and Higgins's self-discrepancy theory relate to how an individual can have low self-esteem if the stigmas conflict with who they want to be. These three theories all relate to how a person feels about himself or herself due to experienced stigma. While stigma relates specifically to feelings of shame and the feelings of failure by not living up to another person's standards, embarrassment is an emotion. Embarrassment is defined as:

> Embarrassment is considered a "self-conscious emotion," and it can have a profoundly negative impact on a person's thoughts or behavior. The embarrassed individual becomes conscious of a real (or imagined) failure to comply with social norms and fears that others won't view them as highly as a result. The ensuing embarrassment may be accompanied by feelings of awkwardness, exposure, shame, guilt, or regret. (*Psychology Today*, 2020)

Thus, while embarrassment may be associated with stigma, the two are not the same thing, and embarrassment may be accompanied by more feelings than just shame. This is why judgment and embarrassment are separated. Examples of embarrassment can be found in 13 of 19 participants. For example, participant 2 states, "It was a little bit embarrassing they would look at what you were buying" (personal communication, July 20, 2020). Participant 2 directly references the word embarrassment in his example, which can also be seen in participant 4's response,

> It made me feel embarrassed. This was back when I couldn't work, I wasn't abusing the benefits I needed, but I felt people that looked at me differently, you are using the government, or a government baby. Why are my taxes going to her Lexus? (personal communication, July 20, 2020)

However, not all examples of embarrassment involve the use of the exact word. Participant 8 is describing her experiences after receiving extra benefits during COVID-19 because her children in a public school receive free lunches, which are then uploaded to a SNAP benefits card. Her example provides a unique insight to COVID-19 and SNAP embarrassment, because she had not been enrolled on SNAP again until COVID-19:

> That is an interesting statement, you know with the free lunch thing with COVID, there is a moment of excitement, OMG I have $600, prior to that our budget for food is $100-$200 for a week. Here is $600 sitting on my table, it is very exciting. We all got ready went to the grocery store, I felt fine, and I knew the moment was coming to pull out that card. I was really excited to maybe get food that we had not been able to get because of the COVID virus. When we get to the cashier, $300 was gone so I pull out the EBT card and immediately my face got hot and I had to pull out the other EBT card. At that moment what it felt like to be totally reliant on food stamps and how shameful to think that if I do not have money for this, I will have to put stuff back which is also embarrassing. (Personal communication, July 10, 2020)

Please note in participant 8's response, the last statement of embarrassment relates to putting stuff back at the grocery checkout, not her SNAP experiences, which is where she discusses shame.

Participant 13 also discusses the embarrassment from having to reenroll on SNAP because of COVID:

> There have been times, now, and I will be honest, even though my husband has been laid off for a period of time. And so when we got it, I was mindful of where I put my card. I do not like people to see my card. Sometimes I swipe my card really quick. People are always making assumptions. To be honest they see a young black woman with kids, they automatically assume think you are food stamps. . . . Now that I am in a place in my life where it does not matter as much to me, sometimes old habits die hard, when I am in a grocery store now, I will still swipe my EBT card fast, because I have been off of SNAP benefits for

many years and just got on them recently because of the pandemic my husband was laid off. (Personal communication, July 27, 2020)

Participant 13 is discussing the embarrassment from using the EBT in the store after being off for many years, and also being an African American woman and the stigma associated with being a SNAP recipient as well as her race. Furthermore, she briefly mentions hiding her EBT card which will be discussed in chapter 7 in avoiding disclosure. These participants provide a brief snapshot into the many examples of individuals feeling embarrassed while enrolled on SNAP.

Unlike the other participants, participant 17, a mixed-race (Hispanic and Middle Eastern descent) cisgender male with no dependents, remembers when he felt being embarrassed to be on SNAP and enrollment as a kid, then receiving the benefits when he is an adult:

> We were kids going in at Walmart; there was a little confrontation that I saw where one guy was talking to another guy, and they fought, etc. Now go buy your food with food stamps. I was like was that insult, wow it is an insult (he did not know what the insult looked like of someone on SNAP as this was his first experience with witnessing that stigma). People that use food stamps do not like to show that they have it, you know. They hide it when they go to the store to block the view of the store. I know subconsciously people in the mind think that other people are looking at them and feel like they do not want to use the benefit. (Personal communication, August 7, 2020)

As many participants felt embarrassed for needing to be enrolled on SNAP, some reported statements of being called lazy, or feeling perceived as being lazy for being enrolled.

Laziness

As with the theme of judging food choices, indicating that a SNAP recipient is lazy also had six participants who reported being called "lazy" or someone insinuated that they are lazy. As with judgment of food choices, individuals feel as though they are being judged as a SNAP recipient as being a lazy person. Participant 7, an African American cisgender female, describes how others look at SNAP recipients, "Probably, I just do not want them looking at me. I think there is a connotation of a black woman that has food stamps. They just do not know. You cannot just not work on and get SNAP" (personal communication, July 23, 2020). She is also describing how race adds to the judgment of being seen as lazy on SNAP.

Similarly, participant 13 describes also being judged for her race and being perceived as lazy because of her enrollment on SNAP, "To be honest they see a young black woman with kids, they automatically assume or think you are on food stamps. They automatically categorize, they automatically think you are lazy" (personal communication, July 27, 2020).

Participant 18, a cisgender Caucasian female, also describes being called "lazy" for being a SNAP recipient,

> I have family members on both sides. While they supported me at the time and knew of my situation, but still would make comments about social programs and how they thought it was I guess used for lazy people. There were also comments about wanting us drug tested before we had access to the benefits. (Personal communication, August 20, 2020)

All of these participants accurately describe the theme of laziness, specifically that SNAP recipients feel they are described as being lazy or do not want to work, when that is not the case. Lastly, while some participants felt embarrassed or judged for being enrolled, some participants further internalized these feelings into deeper feelings of personal failure.

Failure

When compared to the other themes, fewer interviewees (4 of 19) described having a feeling of failure, but their responses indicate a level of emotion they feel about their enrollment. Participant 3 (Caucasian cisgender female) describes how she and her friends feel bad about themselves that they have failed their families because of multigenerational poverty,

> Sometimes because they have similar situations such as the parents think that they are failing their families, and we talk about how the parents do not run their life, and they can do what they want, if they want to afford food that is ok. (Personal communication, July 20, 2020)

Participant 5 (Hispanic cisgender male) also indicates shame and feeling like a failure because of his SNAP enrollment,

> No one wants to admit that they need any help. I felt a lot of I am a failure, I can't provide, I can't stand on my feet. I view myself as very pragmatic. I knew that I needed it. I could have been emotional about it, but I knew that I needed to feed my family. It was a mix of shame, fear. (Personal communication, July 6, 2020)

One final example from participant 19, a cisgender Caucasian female, indicates the feelings of shame and internal stigma from being enrolled, "But the overarching societal shame, and the internal dialogue about needing some financial assistance equating with failure. For the internal dialogue, here I am being a highly educated person and needing food stamps, was constant" (personal communication, August 28, 2020).

All of the participants describe an internalized stigma from their SNAP enrollment that equates failure to them and their families. Though fewer responses than the other themes, internalizing oneself as a failure indicates one of many negative repercussions from being enrolled in the SNAP program and the stigmas many recipients face.

Now that I have described both the statistical results from part 1 and the interview data from part 2, I will bring both sections of the study together by providing more information about what stigma SNAP participants report experiencing.

DIFFERENCES IN STIGMATIZING EXPERIENCES ON SNAP

The total stigma variable from part 1 includes enacted, perceived, felt, internal, and vicarious stigma; the judgment theme from part 2 provides multiple examples of total stigma. Examples of total stigma can be found in the judgment sub-theme, as when participant 1 is describing how her parents told her to just get another job instead of enrolling on SNAP in which verbal judgment is used, causing her to feel stigma, and then not disclose her enrollment to anyone. Participant 12 also provides an example of total stigma when she describes when a lady at Albertson's said, "There goes another one," and she felt shame and embarrassment from the situation and cried in her car. There are many other examples in the interviews that provide examples of stigma with 16 responses in the judgment theme indicating that past and current members all had experiences in which they felt stigma for being enrolled.

Findings in part 1 indicated that people who were migrants or temporary workers, immigrants, had a higher educational attainment, had prior family members who had been enrolled (Generation SNAP), and more members of the household reported having more total stigma. From the 16 participants who reported feeling judged, 5 participants had at least 3 of the variables (31%), 5 had 2 (31%), 2 had 1 (13%), and the rest had none. For example, participant 3 (current) who was a seasonal worker, had some college, and seven members of the household receiving benefits; participant 5 (noncurrent) a seasonal worker, with a master's degree, and a second-generation immigrant; participant 9 (current) a second-generation immigrant, a second-generation

SNAP participant, and four members relying on benefits; and many others with multiple overlapping factors reported examples of judgment and total stigma from being enrolled.

In part 1 there were differences (though sometimes small, depending on the type of stigma) found between current and past recipients of SNAP in all four stigma variables; however, less of a distinguishable difference was found in part 2. While there may not be as distinct a difference between past and current members in the current sample, I did find interesting responses from current members who had been enrolled in the past, and then were off for a period of time and now had to be re-enrolled. Participants 3, 7, and 13 had all been enrolled before and now had re-enrolled because of the COVID-19 pandemic. Participant 13, an African American cisgender female, referenced her past enrollment:

> There have been times, now, and I will be honest, even though my husband has been laid off for a period of time. And so when we got it, I was mindful of where I put my card. . . . Now that I am in a place in my life where it does not matter as much to me, sometimes old habits die hard; when I am in a grocery store now, I will still swipe my EBT card fast, because I have been off of SNAP benefits for many years and just got on them recently because of the pandemic, my husband was laid off. When I wasn't getting, I would go for my sister and pick up her stuff; I didn't want people to judge me about it so I would hide. I still have problems today not wanting people to know about it. My wallet I carry right now, if I open it and can see the EBT card right away. I will move it behind other cards or hide it all together so people cannot see it. (Personal communication, July 27, 2020)

Participant 13 is describing how she thought that she would feel less stigma after having been off a few years but still feels the need to hide her enrollment sometimes.

Similarly, participant 7 also states having issues being reenrolled in the program and dealing with the stigma:

> You know with the free lunch thing with COVID, there is a moment of excitement, OMG I have $600. Prior to that, our budget for food is $100-200 for a week. We all got ready, went to the grocery store, I felt fine, and I knew the moment was coming to pull out that card. I was really excited to maybe get food that we had not been able to get because of the COVID virus. When we get to the cashier, $300 was gone so I pull out the EBT card and immediately my face got hot and I had to pull out the other EBT card. Now I know that the cashier does not care, the little old lady with the Coach bag behind you is staring at you, and the bagger is staring at you, and immediately I thought, "Man, I do not miss being on food stamps." (Personal communication, July 10, 2020)

I highlighted these two examples because I feel that they are discussing how their view of stigma on SNAP has changed from when they had been enrolled the first time to the second time. In fact, participant 7 discussed that when she was first enrolled, she did not feel that much shame from being enrolled, but that it came later, which could help to explain why participant 14, a currently enrolled SNAP recipient, did not feel much stigma from being enrolled. While there may not seem to be many differences between those currently enrolled and past enrolled in reported judgments from the interviews, it highlights that enrollment in SNAP is seen as an overall stigmatizing experience and that even after years of not being enrolled, which was the case for participants 1, 2, 5, 16, 18, and 19, their experiences are still very vivid from their enrollment, even if they are not experiencing them currently.

In the statistical results, data suggests that people are stigmatized while they are enrolled. Specifically, total stigma, past consequences from disclosure, anticipated consequences for disclosure, and disclosure to a specific person were all significant factors that impacted enrollment. Overall the interview data from part 2 supports the statistical findings from part 1 relating to total stigma and SNAP enrollment, specifically that people do experience stigma while enrolled and certain individuals (migrant workers, immigrants, larger households, individuals with higher education attainment, multigenerational SNAP enrollment, etc.) report higher levels of stigma than others. However, the interview data did not support many strong differences between current and past recipients of SNAP. Though I did not provide an in-depth application of SMC to all of the responses relating to stigma (because of the numerous responses relating to stigma and enrollment on SNAP), many of the respondents reporting using SMC tactics such as accepting, reducing offensiveness, avoiding, and denying to improve their chances of hurting their self-esteem from being enrolled; this was not always successful as discussed above where individuals did have feelings of failure, embarrassment, and shame from being "marked." Additional research is needed to go into further detail applying the SMC to the lived experiences of SNAP participants.

However, the effects of stigma do not stop in this chapter alone; the feelings of shame and judgment from being enrolled can then impact the likelihood that participants may disclose to others. As discussed in chapter 3 in the CPM Theory, participants see the disclosure of the SNAP enrollment to others as deeply private information, and because of turbulence, the experiences with stigma and SNAP enrollment may have issues disclosing their enrollment. These issues with disclosing SNAP enrollment will be explored in chapter 7.

Chapter 7

Disclosing SNAP Enrollment Concerns

In chapter 6, I discussed the results relating to total stigma from enrollment on SNAP. Individuals reported having experienced judgment from their enrollment, as well as being accused of committing fraud. As these experiences with stigma and enrollment increased, some participants reported having feelings of embarrassment and failure. All of these feelings and past experiences can lead to concerns disclosing their enrollment to others, as seen in chapter 3 and the CPM Theory and RDT and the chain of discourses. This chapter will provide an in-depth analysis of the statistics and interview data that indicate the impacts of stigma on disclosing one's enrollment to others. I will first go into the statistical data for past consequences from disclosing SNAP enrollment stigma, then anticipated consequences from disclosing SNAP enrollment stigma, and conclude the statistical portion with generalized disclosure concern and disclosure concern to a specific portion.

PAST CONSEQUENCES FROM DISCLOSING SNAP ENROLLMENT STIGMA

After total stigma is discussed in chapter 6, the second primary independent stigma variable formed after the factor analysis is past consequences from disclosing SNAP enrollment stigma. The past consequences from disclosing SNAP enrollment stigma can mean losing friends and family or no longer communicating with individuals based on their SNAP enrollment. To determine how the consequences stigma differed from total stigma, a hierarchical logistic regression was used (table 4.1). The model was significant (Wald χ^2 (9) = 70.60, p = 0.000) with total length, generation SNAP, members of the household, total SES stigma, and total consequences stigma all being significant variables, with migrant status close to significance level. When comparing the goodness of fit scores from the hierarchical logistic regression for total stigma, total consequences stigma has a slightly higher percentage predicted correctly and PRE. Please see table 7.1 for the results from the regression.

As with the prior models, I am providing the maximum and minimum difference of generated predicted probabilities for all significant and close to significance variables to help further explain effect size. Past consequences from disclosing SNAP enrollment stigma had the largest change in predicted probabilities (predicted probabilities [0.53, 0.98] for a change of 0.45) and highest logged odds ratio for individuals who were currently enrolled. Individuals who were currently enrolled had a higher probability of reporting that they had experienced stigma from disclosing their status to friends and families and in turn losing communication. Those who were currently enrolled reported a mean total consequences stigma score of 2.04 (SD = 1.17) compared to those who were no longer enrolled (M = 0.83, SD = 0.81). Of the individuals currently enrolled, 42% reported moderate to the highest score (consequences to disclosure stigma) compared to only 6% of those no longer enrolled. Furthermore, the second largest difference, the number of individuals in the household, was similar to total stigma; the higher the number of individuals in the household, the higher the probability of being currently enrolled (predicted probabilities [0.54, 0.98] for a change of 0.44). While still significant, total length (predicted probabilities [0.81, 0.97] for a change of 0.16) and migrant status (predicted probabilities [0.80, 0.98] for a change of 0.18) had a smaller change in probability for consequences to disclosure than in total stigma. In other words, individuals who were currently enrolled were more likely to report they had been enrolled on the program longer than those who were no longer enrolled, but to a lesser significance level that was found for total stigma. Families who had at least one member of the household that was a migrant or temporary worker had a higher probability of being currently enrolled on SNAP. Furthermore, generation SNAP participant (predicted probabilities [0.69, 0.91] for a negative change of 0.22) and total SES stigma (predicted probabilities [0.74, 0.94] for a negative change of 0.20) had a negative relationship with current enrollment as in total stigma. Participants who were first-generation SNAP users had a lower probability of being enrolled than individuals who had family members who had been enrolled in the past.

To further determine how participants may differ based on the social determinants of health and the past consequences from disclosing SNAP enrollment stigma, a separate OLS regression models analyzed these factors. The model was significant ($F(7,292) = 24.44$, $p = 0.000$). Similar to total stigma, migrant status ($b = 0.16$, $Seb = 0.15$, $\beta = 0.21$), immigrant status ($b = 0.34$,

Table 7.1 Hierarchical Logistic Regression Results for Past Consequence from Disclosing SNAP Enrollment Stigma (DISC-12, IV) and Enrollment Status (DV)

Variable	b	OR	95% CI for b LL	95% CI for b UL	Robust SE b	Pseudo-r^2
Step 1						
Constant	-1.22**	0.29	-2.01	-0.45	0.40	0.27***
Total length	0.19*	1.21	0.04	0.35	0.08	
Migrant status	0.55***	1.73	0.17	0.94	0.20	
Immigrant status	0.64**	1.90	0.18	1.10	0.24	
Education	-0.01	0.99	-0.29	0.28	0.15	
Generation SNAP	-0.39^	0.68	-0.81	0.05	0.22	
Members of the household	0.59***	1.80	0.30	0.89	0.15	
Step 2						
Constant	-1.07*	0.34	-2.27	-0.43	0.47	0.36***
Total length	0.19*	1.21	0.03	0.35	0.08	
Migrant status	0.30^	1.35	0.13	0.83	0.18	
Immigrant status	0.36	1.44	0.06	0.97	0.23	
Education	-0.08	0.92	-0.29	0.27	0.14	
Generation SNAP	-0.74***	0.48	-0.97	-0.06	0.23	
Members of the household	0.65***	1.93	0.27	0.90	0.16	
Total SES[1]	-0.42*	0.66	-0.71	0.02	0.19	
Total Past Consequences Stigma[1]	1.11***	3.03	0.18	1.10	0.24	
Goodness of Fit						
Cragg-Uhler/ Nagelkerke r^2	0.49					
Wald's χ^2 (df = 8)	70.18					
% Predicted Correctly	0.82					
PRE	0.32					

Note: CI = confidence interval; LL = lower limit, UL = upper limit. Pseudo r^2 = McFadden's. The Wald χ^2 is for step 2. PRE = proportion reduction in error or a null model. N = 283. ^p < 0.10, *p < 0.05, **p < 0.01, ***p < 0.001. [1]DISC-12 scale.

Seb = 0.07, β = 0.25), education (b = 0.20, Seb = 0.06, β = 0.18), generation SNAP (b = 0.28, Seb = 0.07, β = 0.16), and members of the household (b = 0.10, Seb = 0.03, β = 0.13) were all significant, but gender was also significant in the model (b = 0.16, Seb = 0.12, β = −0.11). The β scores provide the effect size for all of the variables and the impact it has on past consequences stigma. Once again, immigrant status and migrant status have the largest effect size, meaning they report higher past consequences from disclosing their SNAP enrollment stigma than the other groups.

First, I will provide the means and standard deviations for gender and past consequences from disclosing SNAP enrollment stigma because this was the first model in which gender had a significant relationship. Individuals who reported as cisgender male had slightly higher past consequences from disclosing SNAP enrollment stigma (M = 1.89, SD = 1.28) than cisgender females (M = 1.49, SD = 1.16). Please note the lower means are because participants either scored particularly very high or very low on this variable, meaning participants had very vivid recollection of past severe consequences from disclosing their SNAP enrollment, or they did not.

For past consequences from disclosing SNAP enrollment stigma, those who did not report being or having an individual living in the household who was a migrant or temporary worker had a lower stigma score than in the total stigma category above. Those individuals who lived in the household with an increasing number of migrant or temporary workers reported a higher past consequence from disclosing SNAP enrollment stigma (M = 2.16–2.78, SD = 1.18–1.20) when compared to individuals who did not have a migrant or temporary worker living in the household (M = 0.76, SD = 0.93).

As with total stigma, immigrant status has a significant relationship with past consequences from disclosing SNAP enrollment stigma. Once again, participants who were not third-, second-, or first-generation immigrants had a lower past consequences from disclosure stigma score than those who are immigrants. The results indicate that individuals who reported being a first-generation immigrant (M = 2.56, SD = 1.00), second-generation immigrant (M = 2.28, SD = 1.08), or third-generation immigrant (M = 2.18, SD = 0.98) reported higher stigma from past disclosure of SNAP enrollment than those who were not third generation or closer (M = 0.98, SD = 1.01). Also of note, as a participant moves from being a first-generation to second- and third-generation immigrant, the mean also decreases indicating that first-generation immigrants report the most past consequences from disclosing SNAP enrollment stigma.

When compared to total stigma in chapter 6, educational attainment is a more significant predictor with higher past consequences from disclosing SNAP enrollment stigma. Individuals who had higher educational attainment reported higher past consequences from disclosing SNAP enrollment stigma.

For example, individuals with a high school diploma reported a mean score 0.87(SD = 1.09), whereas individuals with a two-year degree had a mean of 2.10 (SD = 1.16).

Generation SNAP was similar to total stigma. Individuals who had family members who had been enrolled on SNAP in the past reported higher levels past consequences from disclosing SNAP enrollment stigma than those who were first-generation SNAP participants (M = 1.35, SD = 1.23). Specifically, second-generation SNAP users (meaning their parents had been enrolled) had a mean score of 1.99 (SD = 1.23) and third-generation SNAP users had a mean score of 2.20 (SD = 1.07).

Lastly, the number of members of the household is a significant predictor of past consequences of disclosure stigma. Households that reported having more members had higher past consequences from disclosing SNAP enrollment stigma score than smaller households. For example, a household of more than six individuals had a mean score of 2.11 (SD = 1.05), whereas a single individual household reported a mean of 0.57 (SD = 0.57).

Overall, the means were lower for consequences of disclosure stigma; while the significant relationship may exist, participants did not report as large of stigma from consequences of disclosure stigma as the other stigma variables. Earlier consequences of disclosure stigma were described as after disclosing SNAP enrollment, the individuals have lost friends or family who no longer communicate with them. While this may be the case for 33% of the sample that reported having medium-to-high stigma from disclosing their SNAP status, the majority of the sample (42%) reported very little experiences in which friends or family stop communicating with them altogether because of their enrolment, suggesting that strong negative social reactions do happen, and even though not the majority, they are still worth analyzing. Now that I have described briefly the statistical results for past consequences from disclosing SNAP enrollment stigma, I will provide the statistics for the anticipated consequences from disclosing SNAP enrollment stigma.

ANTICIPATED CONSEQUENCES FROM DISCLOSING SNAP ENROLLMENT STIGMA

Anticipated consequences from disclosing SNAP enrollment stigma is different from past consequences because individuals are reported having feelings of anticipating a negative reaction from their disclosure, and thus do not disclose. As in the prior models, a hierarchical logistic regression model is used. The hierarchical logistic regression model for step 2 indicated a significant relationship (Wald χ^2 (8) = 53.67, p = 0.000). The results from the hierarchical logistic regression model are depicted in table 7.2.

Table 7.2 Hierarchical Logistic Regression Results for Anticipated Consequences from Disclosing SNAP Enrollment Stigma (DISC-12, IV) and Enrollment Status (DV)

Variable	b	OR	95% CI for b LL	95% CI for b UL	Robust SE b	Pseudo-r^2
Step 1						0.27^{***}
Constant	-1.29^{**}	0.28	-2.07	-0.50	0.40	
Total length	0.20^{*}	1.22	0.04	0.35	0.08	
Migrant status	0.54^{**}	1.72	0.17	0.92	0.19	
Immigrant status	0.64^{**}	1.90	0.18	1.10	0.24	
Education	0.01	1.00	-0.28	0.29	0.15	
Generation SNAP	$-0.37^{\wedge}$	0.69	-0.80	0.06	0.22	
Members of the household	0.59^{***}	1.80	0.29	0.89	0.15	
Step 2						0.28^{***}
Constant	-1.18^{*}	0.31	-2.07	-0.28	0.46	
Total length	0.19^{*}	1.21	0.03	0.35	0.08	
Migrant status	0.55^{*}	1.73	0.18	0.94	0.19	
Immigrant status	0.64^{*}	1.89	0.17	1.10	0.24	
Education	-0.001	1.00	-0.28	0.27	0.14	
Generation SNAP	$-0.42^{\wedge}$	0.66	-0.86	0.03	0.23	
Members of the household	0.57^{***}	1.46	0.25	0.88	0.16	
Total SES stigma[1]	-0.39^{*}	0.68	-0.78	-0.01	0.19	
Total Anticipated stigma[1]	0.45^{*}	1.57	0.06	0.84	0.20	
Goodness of Fit						
Cragg-Uhler/Nagelkerke r^2	0.40					
Wald's χ^2 (df = 8)	53.67					
% Predicted Correctly	0.80					
PRE	0.26					

Note: CI = confidence interval; LL = lower limit, UL = upper limit. Pseudo r^2 = McFadden's. The Wald χ^2 is for step 2. PRE = Proportion reduction in error or a null model. N = 279. $^{\wedge}p < 0.10$, $^{*}p < 0.05$, $^{**}p<0.01$, $^{***}p < 0.001$. [1]DISC-12 scale.

The significant factors from the model are similar to both total stigma and past consequences from disclosing SNAP enrollment stigma with total length, migrant status, immigrant status, members of the household, total SES stigma, and anticipated consequences from disclosing SNAP enrollment all being significant. Generation SNAP was also close to significance level (p = 0.07).

To explain effect size, I am providing the odds ratio for anticipated consequences from disclosing SNAP enrollment stigma, and the minimum and maximum probabilities for all significant variables. For anticipated consequences from disclosing SNAP enrollment stigma, for every one-unit change, there is 0.45 increase in the log-odds ratio that an individual is currently enrolled. In addition to the logged odd ratio, I include the minimum and maximum predicted probabilities for anticipated consequences from disclosing SNAP enrollment and current enrollment and the significant variables.

When compared to the two models of stigma, anticipated consequences from disclosing SNAP enrollment is the weakest in terms of the change in predicted probabilities (predicted probabilities [0.65, 0.92] for a change of 0.27). The strongest variable in the model is members of the household (more members of the household a higher probability of being currently enrolled compared to those who are not currently enrolled, predicted probabilities [0.55, 0.97] for a change of 0.42); second is the total anticipated consequences from disclosing SNAP enrollment. Those who were currently enrolled had a higher probability of identifying higher levels of anticipated consequences from disclosing SNAP enrollment from SNAP than those not enrolled. Those currently enrolled reported a mean anticipated consequences from disclosing SNAP enrollment score of 2.13 (SD = 1.59) compared to those who were no longer enrolled (M = 1.59, SD = 1.09). Of the individuals currently enrolled, 54% reported high to the highest amount of anticipated consequences from disclosing SNAP enrollment compared to 28% of those no longer enrolled. Of all of the stigma variables, anticipated consequences from disclosing SNAP enrollment have the highest number of individuals reporting moderate-to-high stigma but the weakest relationship.

The other significant variables and their predicted probabilities are total length (predicted probabilities [0.77, 0.96] for a total change of 0.19), migrant status (predicted probabilities [0.70, 0.99] for a total change of 0.29), immigrant status (predicted probabilities [0.75, 0.95] for a change of 0.20), generation of SNAP use (predicted probabilities [0.74, 0.86] for a negative change of 0.13), and SES stigma (predicted probabilities [0.70, 0.93] for a change of 0.23).

To help provide more context for the social determinants found in the model and anticipated consequences from disclosure, a second OLS regression model was used. The model was significant ($F_{(5,295)} = 13.69$, p = 0.000). The only two significant variables in the model for anticipated consequences from disclosing SNAP enrollment stigma were educational attainment (b = 0.16, Seb = 0.06, β = 0.16) and members of the household (b = 0.17, Seb = 0.04, β = 0.23) with generation SNAP being close to significance level (p = 0.046, b = 0.15, Seb = 0.08, β = 0.10). The β scores indicate that the number of members of the household had the largest impact on total stigma.

For educational attainment, individuals who reported higher educational attainment (M = 2.32, SD = 1.24) also reported higher levels of anticipated consequences from disclosing SNAP enrollment stigma compared to those who had less. Individuals who had a high school diploma reported a mean score of 1.42 (SD = 1.24) compared to individuals with a two-year degree (M = 2.49, SD = 1.07).

Next, as with all other models, the number of members of the household is a significant variable. The more individuals relying on SNAP benefits living in one household, the higher reported anticipated consequences from disclosing SNAP enrollment stigma. For example, a family of six or greater had a mean score of 2.55 (0.73), whereas a single individual has a mean score of 1.4(SD = 1.65).

Lastly, I have included generation SNAP because of how close the variable was to significance level. As with all models, individuals who had prior family members who had also been enrolled on SNAP reported higher anticipated consequences from disclosing SNAP enrollment stigma than those who were first generation (M = 1.99, SD = 1.23). Third-generation SNAP participants reported the most anticipated consequences from disclosing their SNAP enrollment with a mean of 2.5 (SD = 1.06), whereas second-generation SNAP participants had a mean of 2.37 (SD = 1.17).

Though not as mean significant variables as the prior two models, anticipated consequences from disclosing SNAP enrollment stigma has overall higher means than past consequences from disclosing SNAP enrollment stigma with 48% of the sample indicating medium-to-high reported levels of anticipated consequences from disclosing SNAP enrollment stigma.

In addition to the past and anticipated consequences from disclosing SNAP enrollment stigma, the original factor analysis indicated that there is also a generalized SNAP enrollment disclosure concern and concern for disclosing to a specific person

GENERALIZED SNAP ENROLLMENT DISCLOSURE CONCERN

To determine how generalized SNAP enrollment disclosure concern differs based on enrollment status, a hierarchical logistic regression was used; however, for generalized SNAP enrollment disclosure concern, there was not a significant difference across enrollment (p = 0.80) whereas the model itself was significant ($\chi^2 = 86.65$, p = 0.000). The model included the same significant variables as in prior models: total length enrolled, migrant status, immigrant status, and members of the household. The mean score for generalized SNAP enrollment disclosure concern for the individuals who were currently enrolled was 2.31 (SD = 1.03) and 2.03 (SD = 1.13) for those no longer enrolled, but this difference was not significant after controlling for the sociodemographic variables. Because generalized SNAP enrollment disclosure concern was the primary IV in this model, I will not further discuss the generalized disclosure concern variable.

An important note about generalized SNAP enrollment disclosure concern is this variable describes the ability to keep their enrollment status a secret and the riskiness of telling about their enrollment. While generalized SNAP enrollment disclosure concern was not associated with a particular person, I also performed a hierarchical logistic regression model to determine if disclosing SNAP enrollment was more of an issue with a specific person than asking about disclosure concern in general.

The second hierarchical logistic regression model for disclosure concerns is associated with how individuals who are enrolled in SNAP may have concerns for disclosing their SNAP enrollment to specific individuals. The results from these two models are shown in table 7.3. The second model was significant ($\chi2 = 60.90$, p = 0.000).

Similar to prior models, total length, migrant status, immigrant status, members of the household, and concern for disclosing SNAP enrollment to a specific person stigma were all significant variables in the model with generation SNAP being close to significance level. To explain the effect size for the variables, I include the minimum and maximum probability for disclosure concerns to a specific source and current enrollment.

Participants who reported having an individual living in the house as a migrant or temporary worker had a higher probability of being enrolled currently (predicted probabilities [0.71, 0.99] for a change of 0.28). Individuals who were currently enrolled also had a higher probability of being an immigrant or descended from immigrants (predicted probabilities [0.75, 0.95] for a change of 0.20).

Generation SNAP was also a negative relationship as seen in other models; individuals currently enrolled were more likely to be from multiple generation of SNAP participants (predicted probabilities [0.75. 0.87] for a negative change of 0.12). The variable with highest change in the minimum and maximum probability, members in the household, has the strongest association with current enrollment (predicted probabilities [0.55, 0.97] for a change 0.42). Participants were more probable to be currently enrolled if they had more individuals living in their household who used benefits. Lastly,

Table 7.3 Hierarchical Logistic Regression Results for Concern for Disclosing SNAP Enrollment to a Specific Person (Wright et al., IV) and Enrollment Status (DV)

Variable	b	OR	95% CI for b		Robust SE b	Pseudo-r^2
			LL	UL		
Step 1						
Constant	-1.19*	0.30	-1.98	-0.41	0.40	0.26***
Total length	0.19*	1.20	0.03	0.34	0.20	
Migrant status	0.54*	1.71	0.15	0.92	0.20	
Immigrant status	0.64*	1.89	0.18	1.10	0.23	
Education	-0.006	1.00	-0.29	0.28	0.14	
Generation SNAP	-0.38^	0.68	-0.81	0.05	0.22	
Members of the household	0.58***	1.80	0.29	0.88	0.15	
Step 2						
Constant	-1.18*	0.31	-2.10	-0.27	0.47	0.27***
Total length	0.17*	1.19	0.01	0.33	0.08	
Migrant status	0.50*	1.65	0.13	0.87	0.19	
Immigrant status	0.61*	1.84	0.14	1.07	0.24	
Education	-0.002	1.00	-0.28	0.28	0.14	
Generation SNAP	-0.39^	0.67	-0.84	0.04	0.22	
Members of the household	0.57***	1.76	0.26	0.88	0.16	
Total SES Stigma[1]	0.77	0.95	-0.60	0.08	0.18	
Total concern for disclosing to a specific person[2]	1.41*	0.92	-0.002	0.69	0.18	
Goodness of Fit						
Cragg-Uhler/Nagelkerke r^2	0.39					
% Predicted correctly	0.80					
PRE	0.27					

Note: CI = confidence interval; LL = lower limit, UL = upper limit. Pseudo r^2 = Mcfadden's. The Wald χ^2 is for step 2. PRE = proportion reduction in error or a null model. N = 279. ^p < 0.10, *p < 0.05, **p < 0.01, ***p < 0.001. [1]DISC-12 scale; [2]Wright et al. (2007) stigma scale.

individuals who were currently enrolled had a higher probability of concern for disclosing their SNAP enrollment to others compared to those who were no longer currently enrolled (predicted probabilities [0.71, 0.90] for a change of 0.19); however, the probability is still high indicating that those no longer enrolled still have some concern for revealing their SNAP enrollment to others.

Though not as strong a predictor as prior models, total disclosure concerns sources are still an essential factor in my study. Importantly, while total disclosure concerns and total disclosure concerns sources both are specifically related to an instrument that measures disclosure concerns, both anticipated consequences from disclosing SNAP enrollment and past consequences from disclosing SNAP enrollment stigma have many elements that are related to disclosure of one's SNAP enrollment regardless of the specific label used in prior studies (not specifically labeled a communicative component).

As with anticipated and past consequences, a separate regression that looked at how the different sociodemographic variables (social determinants of health) may impact who an individual interprets disclosure concerns about SNAP enrollment was used. The model was significant ($F (6,294) = 10.34$, $p = 0.000$).

As with most of the earlier models, migrant status ($b = 0.08$, $Se_b = 0.04$, $\beta = 0.11$), immigrant status ($b = 0.22$, $Se_b = 0.07$, $\beta = 0.19$) , education ($b = 0.13$, $Se_b = 0.06$, $\beta = 0.13$), and members of the household ($b = 0.11$, $Se_b = 0.03$, $\beta = 0.16$) were all significant, with generation SNAP being close to significance ($p = 0.08$). The β scores indicated effect size. Immigrant status followed by members of the household benefiting from SNAP have the largest effect size on disclosure concerns to specific individuals.

Specific for migrant status, the same relationship exists as in prior models. Of all the important independent variables which have been discussed, disclosure concern for a specific person or source is the first in which a mean has been at a three (3) or higher, indicating a moderate level of high concern for disclosing SNAP enrollment to a specific person. For migrant or temporary workers, as more individuals in a household are migrant workers or temporary workers, the higher the disclosure concern when compared to others who have fewer members who are or who are not migrant or temporary workers. In other words, if a household has multiple members who are migrant or temporary workers, that is a high amount of disclosure concern to tell others (regardless of who) about their SNAP enrollment. For example, the mean score for having at least three members of the household that are migrant or temporary workers is 3.11 ($SD = 0.78$), compared to households that did not have any migrant or temporary workers ($M = 1.74$, $SD = 1.10$). This indicates that migrant and temporary workers are highly concerned with whom they disclose their enrollment status.

Additionally, immigrant status is similar to all of the previous models, but not at the level of fear for disclosure as with migrant status. There is a substantial difference between those who do not have a family member who has immigrated to the United States (M = 1.72, SD = 1.11) compared to a first-generation immigrant (M = 2.83, SD = 0.82). The disclosure concern score for first generation is almost at the moderate or agree with high levels of stigma. Whereas third generation (M = 2.6, SD = 1.07) and second generation (M = 2.49, SD = 0.96) are still higher than most of the other immigrant status significance levels found in the other models. Indicating there is a moderate-to-high level of concern for disclosing their SNAP enrollment to specific individuals.

After migrant and immigration status is educational attainment. As educational attainment increases, so does the concern for disclosing SNAP enrollment to others. Specifically, individuals with a two-year degree report a mean score of 2.54(SD = 0.96), compared to a high school graduate with 1.57(SD = 1.10).

The last significant variable, the number of members of the household, is the most significant as in many of the prior models. As a household size increases, the concern for disclosure of SNAP status increases. The largest increase is from two individuals who use the SNAP benefits to more than three. A family of more than six individuals report a mean score of 2.44 (SD = 0.73) compared to a single individual with a score of 1.39 (SD = 0.91)/

The final and only variable that was close to significance level, generation SNAP, will be briefly discussed. The difference across generations on SNAP is not as strong as in some of the earlier models. As individuals report more past family members who have been enrolled (M = 2.43, SD = 0.87), there is a slight increase in disclosure concerns when compared to first-generation SNAP participants (M = 2.03, SD = 1.17).

In addition to the total stigma discussed in chapter 6, past consequences from SNAP enrollment stigma, anticipated consequences from SNAP enrollment disclosure stigma, and disclosure concern to a specific person all had significant factors that impacted current enrollment as well as social demographic factors (social determinants of health) that impacted the severity of the perceived stigma. In addition to the statistical results for disclosure concerns and SNAP enrolment, avoiding discussion of SNAP enrollment theme found in the interview data is one of the most mentioned themes in all 19 participants.

AVOIDING DISCUSSION OF SNAP ENROLLMENT INTERVIEW THEME

Sixteen of the 19 participants reported wanting to avoid discussion of their SNAP enrollment with others. Avoiding discussion relates to the concern for disclosing SNAP enrollment to a specific person stigma reported in the results from the first survey, specifically that individuals often choose not to talk about the SNAP enrollment. Part 2 findings indicate that lack of specificity in the source of disclosure concern found in part 1 could be from the varying ways in which individuals avoid discussion of their enrollment. Avoiding discussion has three sub-themes: avoiding disclosure to family or friends, avoiding discussion to the generalized other, and hiding the EBT card in the grocery store.

Avoiding Disclosure to a Specific Individual

Eleven of 19 participants reported wanting to avoid discussion of their SNAP enrollment with a specific individual such as participant 10, a Caucasian cisgender female, "Yes, we do not talk about it at all. We keep it to ourselves. Hide it from family and friends. We choose to hide it from family and friends" (personal communication, July 21, 2020). Participant 10 chose to not tell anyone about her enrollment but points out that she chose to hide it from family and friends. Similarly, participant 3, a Caucasian 33-year-old cisgender female, also felt the need to not disclose to a particular family member, "We just do not talk about that to her or her family members so she doesn't have any reason to bring it up. To avoid the conversation altogether or the people that know her" (personal communication, July 7, 2020). Participant 19, a 47-year-old cisgender female, also reported not wanting to disclose to a specific group of people, "Especially clients for sure, I did not go around broadcasting to anybody" (personal communication, August 28, 2020).

Furthermore, participant 13 (an African American cisgender female) also shares how she has hidden her enrollment from others:

> Yes, I have hid it. Co-workers, even sometimes everybody. There have been times when not even my close family knew. Still going back to the fact that you want people to form opinions on you based on the enrollment. This more recent enrollment while my husband is off job, my coworker who is just so stereotypical she is trying but just not there, she mentioned something that her mother-in-law receives food stamps, but I have never mentioned to her that we have went and applied. (Personal communication, July 27, 2020)

Participant 13 feels the need to have to keep her enrollment a secret from her coworkers, even though the coworker's mother-in-law also receives benefits. For participant 13, the stigma from being a SNAP recipient and fearing being stereotyped for being enrolled is memorable.

Avoiding Disclosure to the Generalized Other

The avoiding disclosure to the generalized other sub-theme is when individuals do not name a person to whom they choose to not disclose but to just society at large. Eleven of 19 participants mentioned not wanting to disclose to anybody in general.

Unlike participants 3, 10, and 19, participant 5, a Hispanic cisgender male, more generally does not want to disclose his SNAP enrollment, "Yes, I still feel the need to hide it from others, still I will never tell it to anyone else except for this interview" (personal communication, July 6, 2020).

Participant 1, a 38-year-old African American cisgender female, also avoids discussion of SNAP more generally:

> I grew up in a very, very, very poor household. But my parents are very prideful and would rather work 4–5 jobs than to get on food stamps. Which would probably have helped us growing up, they chose not to even though they definitely qualified, they made minimum wage. We had a large household. I got on food stamps when we were in college, that is when I utilized it. No one really knew that I was on it, so I didn't really feel stigmatized while I was on it. (Personal communication, July 7, 2020)

While participant 1 shares that she may not have felt stigmatized while she was enrolled, she felt the need to not disclose her enrollment or at least chose not to share to others for reasons based on her family history/attitudes.

Avoiding Disclosure of the EBT Card

The avoiding disclosure of the EBT card sub-theme relates to individuals who feel the need to keep others from seeing their EBT card in stores. These are individuals who do not wish to disclose their SNAP enrollment by showing other people in the grocery store that they have an EBT card. Six participants out of 19 mentioned hiding their EBT card in stores. For example, participant 7, an African American college student states,

> The Louisiana food stamp card is hideous and very obvious; I usually use self-checkout majority of the time. Never to my face, all of the people I talk to tell me to my face, help me apply to SNAP. . . . No, I pick who I tell. If I feel they

will not react right, I just will not let them know. I would not tell them. They do not need to know how I buy food. I do have rich friends, by rich I mean upper-middle class. They just will not know; when we go grocery shopping, I make sure that they are somewhere else when I am self-checkout. They do not need to know everything. (Personal communication, July 10, 2020)

Participant 7 is hiding her card when she mentions that she purposefully uses a means of checking out her groceries so that the cashier does not see the card. She also is careful who she uses the EBT card in front of, specifically to avoid being seen differently because of her using the card in a grocery store. Similarly, participant 9, a Caucasian woman, also reports hiding her card at the store:

Mostly when I go to the store. The Dollar Store you actually have to say that I have food stamps, the credit or debit that is when you start to get the dirty looks. Sometimes you can hide the card when you swipe it, but if you have to announce that you have food stamps, God forbid that I am dressed for work, and I have a nice shirt on and all of that stuff. The looks will get way worse. I am dressed all nice, the looks get worse. (Personal communication, July 21, 2020)

The statistical results did not indicate a substantial difference among the sources of disclosure concern (family, friends, strangers, etc.), suggesting that people chose a variety of people to not tell their SNAP enrollment because of specific reasons. The findings from the interviews suggest that individuals may avoid disclosure of their SNAP enrollment to a wide variety of individuals, a generalized other, and their EBT card in grocery stores. Overall, the theme of avoiding discussion or disclosure is important in terms of social support and stigma and SNAP enrollment and will be discussed further in chapter 6.

To help provide further context for the breadth of individuals to whom participants avoid disclosure, I have included a word cloud (figure 7.1) that includes the main sources for whom participants reported having the most disclosure concern stigma. While three participants said no one, many name-specific relationships to them such as family and significant others, but also a generalized other such as strangers.

IMPLICATIONS FOR THE DIFFERENT TYPES OF DISCLOSURE CONCERN STIGMA

As seen in the interview themes, SNAP participants often feel some concern for disclosing their enrollment to others. From the responses, it is clear that

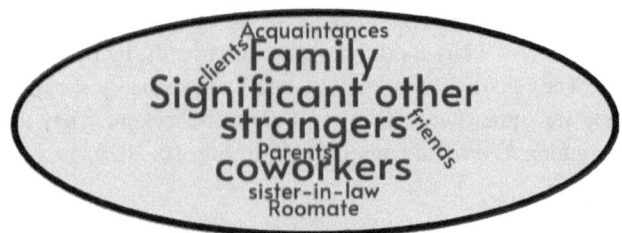

Figure 7.1 Concern for Disclosing SNAP Enrollment to a Specific Person Examples.
Source: Created by the author.

the act of disclosing such private information is not a cut and dry process, but a complex and often hard decision to make based on numerous factors, specifically in terms of past consequences from disclosing stigma, anticipated stigma from disclosing to others, and concern for disclosing SNAP enrollment to a specific person.

Past Consequences from Disclosing SNAP Enrollment

In the interview process for past consequences from disclosing SNAP enrollment stigma, only one participant felt he/she had lost family members because of enrollment (participant 12), but several individuals reported they had decided to not inform their friends or family, which relates more toward concern for disclosing SNAP enrollment to a specific person stigma. Thus, in the 19 participants, there was not support for the past consequences from disclosing SNAP enrollment stigma found in the surveys. However, in chapter 4, I noted that this was a highly divisive category—one had either had this experience or not. Because many participants reported having strong social support circles, whether through friends or family, it was not surprising to see only one participant mention that he or she had less contact with family members.

Next, several sub-themes from chapter 6 also relate to feelings of fear or anticipation of a negative reaction to disclosing one's SNAP enrollment.

Anticipated Consequences from Disclosing SNAP Enrollment

Three sub-themes relate to the feelings of how anticipating consequences from disclosing SNAP enrollment could impact one's personal identity by worrying about reactions from others, and then choosing to not disclose enrollment to others: embarrassment ($n = 10$), failure ($n = 6$), and laziness ($n = 7$). As in the statistical findings, the interviews reflect that fewer participants experience those feelings of anticipated consequences from disclosing SNAP enrollment stigma than total stigma and concern for disclosing SNAP enrollment to a specific person stigma. Regardless, several participants match the factors found in the survey data that increased the level of anticipated consequences from disclosing SNAP enrollment stigma: higher educational attainment, prior family members that had been enrolled on SNAP, and larger dependent households. Participant 19 (a second-generation SNAP recipient with 5dependents) reported experiencing all three themes that reflect anticipated consequences from disclosing SNAP enrollment stigma, and participant 13 (a second-generation SNAP recipient with 7 dependents) identified both embarrassment for being enrolled and a fear of being considered lazy. Participants 8 (third-generation SNAP recipient with 5 dependents), 12 (second-generation SNAP recipient with a doctorate degree, and 4 dependents), 3 (with some college and 7 dependents), and 2 (second-generation SNAP recipient, a master's degree, and four dependents) all reported having felt embarrassed for being enrolled, indicating that while fewer in number than the other types of stigma, anticipated consequences from disclosing SNAP enrollment stigma does occur and can be more impactful for individuals with multiple different levels of intersectionality.

Lastly, concern for disclosing SNAP enrollment to a specific person is clearly shown in the avoiding discussion theme in the interview as well as the statistical data.

Concern for Disclosing SNAP Enrollment to a Specific Person Stigma

As with the statistical results, many participants did not seem to have a preference to whom they were most concerned with disclosing their SNAP enrollment unless there was a history of judgment; thus, the source did not matter as much as did the feeling of needing to hide enrollment. Two sub-themes from chapter 4 reflect this fear of disclosing one's SNAP enrollment due to the fear of judgment or an actual response, avoiding discussion, and hiding the card/enrollment. As far as differences between current and past members, several past members shared with me that they initially did not even want to do the interview because their feelings from being enrolled were so strong, as in participant 7,

> Yeah, I do not like to talk about it. I was even hesitant to do the interview honestly, because it is something I want to put behind me. It is something that I am not proud of it, and it is embarrassing. It is also what I had to do; by the grace of God, we are not there anymore. (Personal communication, July 10, 2020)

Participant 5 also shares,

Not that I am aware of, I still have not disclosed that to anyone. Other than receiving disaster benefits from the flood of 2016. We got on that because everyone was on that, there was no stigma because it was a unique situation. Everyone knew that everyone was on it. (Personal communication, July 6, 2020)

Similarly, participant 10 also did not like sharing information about her experiences enrolled on SNAP:

NO (emphatically), I never talk about it (SNAP enrollment) . . . I do not know if I want to talk about this; we do not talk about this to anyone. It is not like telling a stranger this information, 'cause we know you, and I know there is no judgment coming from you. It is not easy, it is not an easy application process, it is not an easy program to be on. I guess if you have never been on it, you do not understand. (Personal communication, July 21, 2020)

Those participants who were not currently enrolled were the individuals who were not as comfortable sharing their experiences on SNAP and also those who told me they did not like conducting the interviews. This is not to say that individuals who were currently enrolled were not concerned with disclosing to others, but they were more comfortable disclosing to me. As a reminder, 15 participants mentioned avoiding discussions about SNAP with others and 11 noted hiding their enrollment.

In addition to the differences between current and past members, as with the total stigma findings, there were also several individuals who had multiple significant factors for disclosure concerns. Statistical findings indicated that individuals who were migrant or temporary workers, an immigrant, had higher educational attainment, family members who had been prior members of SNAP (generation SNAP) and had larger household reported more disclosure concern stigma. Several interviewees had multiple factors influencing their disclosure concern stigma: participant 3 (seasonal worker, some college, and 7 dependents), participant 5 (a seasonal worker, master's degree, and a second-generation immigrant), participant 7 (some college degree and a third-generation SNAP recipient), participant 8 (third-generation SNAP recipient and 5 dependents), participant 2 (master's degree, second-generation SNAP recipient, and 4 dependents), and many others. Overall, a diverse pool of interviewees yielded individuals who had many background factors that impact their fear of disclosing their SNAP enrollment to others. Furthermore, the results from this chapter highlighted a concern that I have for participants who have been enrolled or are currently enrolled on SNAP, which is, do these individuals who have strong concerns for disclosing their SNAP enrollment not have access to strong social support systems? Social support will be discussed in chapter 8.

CONCLUSION

Overall, the results from the interview reflect the statistical results, except for small differences between individuals who are currently enrolled and past enrolled. Individuals with more than one demographic factor tend to have more instances of reporting experiences involving stigma on SNAP. The 19 participants reflect the importance of considering intersectionality among participants when looking at experiences of SNAP recipients because as an individual has multiple demographic factors interacting, the person is reporting more stigma from SNAP than other participants. The recorded responses about the three stigma variables indicate how stigmatizing the enrollment of SNAP is for most individuals, and sometimes how the feelings of stigma can then impact one's internal feelings of identity and stop individuals from disclosing their enrollment to others and possibly impact the social support received. However, the stigma variables alone do not offer a complete picture of the experiences of SNAP participants; the second research question will apply the statistical results and interview of findings from social support in chapter 8.

Chapter 8

Social Support from Family and Friends and SNAP Enrollment

In chapters 5, 6, and 7, I discussed how enrollment on SNAP can have negative unintended consequences such as dissatisfaction with the program, stigma, and fear of disclosing to others. However, in this chapter, I will discuss how social support can help alleviate some of these problems as long as the support is positive and does not add to the stigmatizing effects of enrollment. Please note that all of the information presented in this chapter is from the interview process; no questions pertaining to social support were asked in the statistical portion of the study. In the interview process, people reported having received some element of social support, whether positive or negative, from both friends and family members.

SOCIAL SUPPORT

During the interview process, 17 of the 19 recipients reported receiving some type of social support—informational, tangible, esteem, and emotional. Though all four are present, there did not seem to be a consistent theme on what was more important to someone; in fact, the source of the support seemed to be more salient to participants. Thus, there are four primary sub-themes: supportive friends, unsupportive friends, supportive family, and unsupportive family. In addition to the four primary sub-themes, there are combinations of all four.

Supportive Friends

Eleven interviewees of the 17 that discussed having some type of social support mentioned having supportive friends in their social circles while they were enrolled in SNAP. An example of supportive friends can be found in participant 7's (a 20-year-old African American cisgender female) response about receiving social support:

> I would say yes, I was living off of soda and snacks, I had no food. I had friends at the time that would buy me food. I get taken to the grocery store. My friends will cook for me, and I will cook for them. Tangible is a big yes. I had a friend gave me $50 because you need to get the food, his friend had given it to him, so we were passing the same money for food. Tangible the most of the three. They are supportive of just talking about, or I help others get on it. (Personal communication, July 10, 2020)

Participant 7 is describing that while she was enrolled in SNAP, her friends were providing her with food and money to help, specifically while she is in college.

Participant 3, a 30-year-old Caucasian cisgender female with seven dependents, relates to the question about who do you feel judgment from, and she responded not friends because they are also poor and have had experiences with SNAP in the past,

> No, not friends because most of them are in the same situation as we are so it is not a problem. I have helped most of them get enrolled on SNAP and back on their feet, so most of those friends are very understanding. (Personal communication, July 7, 2020)

Furthermore, participant 13 (an African American cisgender female) states that she uses humor with some of her friends to help her through the judgment:

> I told her besides even if I did I would not sell them to you I want it all for myself! LOL! The fact that she had the audacity to just come to me to assume. She assumes that I have 7 kids I was on food stamps. Then she was like Oh save my number this is my new number? I thought Oh sure I am definitely going to save your number now that you insulted me. Then she asked me "Do you know of anyone that is selling" I have a mutual girlfriend that I had to call to tell her about the story (we both know her). (Personal communication, July 27, 2029)

Participant 13 is describing an incident in which she was being asked to commit fraud and felt insulted so she called her friend that also knew the woman and discussed the situation with her. All of these responses highlight that positive social support from friends can help individuals through their stigmatizing experiences while enrolled on SNAP.

Unsupportive Friends

When compared to the number of individuals who reported having supportive friends, only one person, participant 7, reported having an unsupportive friend while enrolled on SNAP:

> Acquaintances who have been known to side or mention things about people who (are) on welfare, or they mention something slick about SNAP now. I know I can't trust you I do not want you to take me to the grocery store. I do not have a car, so I rely on my roommate to take me to the store, and she doesn't even know that I have food stamps. Not that I do not trust her, but she is top level middle-class family. They took us to some super expensive restaurant; this is why I will not tell you because you do not understand. They are sweet people but I will not bring it up. (Personal communication, July 10, 2020)

In this example, participant 7 is describing to whom she has chosen to not disclose her enrollment, specifically her friend that is also her roommate, because she is scared of the judgment that she may have on her since her roommate's family is wealthy. However, it is revealing to me that individuals who are enrolled on SNAP, both current and past, positively discuss their friends as important sources of social support if they have shared their status with them.

Supportive Family

While many of the participants reported supportive friends, 15 of 17 reported having some type of supportive family members while enrolled in SNAP. Participant 5's (36-year-old Hispanic cisgender male with four dependents) response helps describe what a supportive family member provides:

> No, I did talk to my father and my wife, we discussed at length, about how we can budget the money. With my dad, we talked about the situation why I needed it that I would not be able to provide for my family. The whole nine yards with that. He would help us out when we go out to the grocery store, I would use those funds to help both, and provide some kind of benefits to him as well. Which we were going to eat anyway so we were still using it correctly. (Personal communication, July 6, 2020).

Participant 5 is describing how both his father and wife helped provide emotional support as well as tangible support while he was enrolled on SNAP.

Similarly, participant 10, a Caucasian cisgender female with four dependents, highlighted support from her parents as well,

> I think it is great. I do not know if I want to talk about this; we do not talk about this to anyone. It is not easy, it is not an easy application process, it is not an easy program to be on. I guess if you have never been on it, you do not understand. My mom was very understanding. (Personal communication, July 21, 2020)

She is highlighting how being enrolled in the program is stigmatizing, but that her mother helped them get through their time enrolled.

Participant 12, a cisgender, Caucasian female, agrees with participant 10 with the support of a mother and dealing with the stigma while enrolled:

> Oh yeah. I would call my mom in tears, and she would be like why are you letting these people get to you and you do not even know them. I said I don't know, it is just so embarrassing to be in the line at the grocery store, but they always sigh or make some type of snide comment. It is just so hurtful. You know my family had been so supportful with everything and helped us out with diapers. And we were very poor. (Personal communication, August 6, 2020).

As with supportive friends, there is evidence that positive social support from family members can help them through their enrollment, but not all participants have a supportive family structure, or they may have some supportive family members but not all.

Unsupportive Family

Fewer participants reported having unsupportive family members, but of those eight, the responses were often repeated as in this response from participant 1, an African American cisgender female,

> My family was like why don't you get another job? Well, I was already in school, and I had a job. I didn't want to. The school I was going to definitely wasn't easy; you had to do a work study because I went to a tuition free school. (Personal communication, July 10, 2020)

Shortly after describing that her parents would criticize her and tell her she should get another job, she comments,

> From them especially lol, just them telling me why don't you just get a second job, you do not need to get SNAP, just get another second job. They didn't treat me any different. Why do you need to get on food stamps? That was mainly it. They were over it after they told me their opinion about it. I couldn't talk to them much about it after that. Now, I was like, "Why did y'all not get on it?

We qualified for it; we would not have been so hungry growing up." (Personal communication, July 10, 2020)

Participant 1 also notes that her parents are the main ones to whom she was most concerned to disclose her SNAP enrollment.

A similar response about unsupportive family can be observed from participant 4, a cisgender, Caucasian female with seven dependents, who is specifically highlighting the lack of support from her sister-in-law,

> My sister-in-law is very against it; her and her husband are the only ones that have something negative to say about using it. We just do not talk about that to her or her family members so she doesn't have any reason to bring it up. To avoid the conversation altogether or the people that know her. (Personal communication, July 20, 2020)

Immediately following this discussion, she states, "I do not think so, she doesn't get to make decisions on my enrollment. She is not supporting my family so she can move along" (personal communication, July 20, 2020).

Another example of an unsupportive family member comes from participant 8, a Caucasian cisgender female with more than five dependents:

> I can remember when I was younger and a foster kid and a teen mom, and the foster dad that I had, and I needed to get groceries so I asked him to take to me to the store, and he was very hesitant to do so. So I asked him if we take the SNAP card and a list of groceries and go yourself if you would rather do that. He was like absolutely not, I will not be seen with that card. It was obvious that he was ashamed to be using something like that. (Personal communication, July 10, 2020)

Lastly, participant 11 (a cisgender, Caucasian male) reported feeling ashamed and made fun of by extended family:

> My wife's family know how to work the system they suggested that we get on SNAP even though I did not want to and I was ashamed, they mocked me and said I was riding the disability train because of my injury. They make me uncomfortable that they know our financial business even though I do not want them to know anything. (Personal communication, July 23, 2020)

All of these are examples of individuals who strictly reported only having unsupportive family members, not combinations of supportive family members. Furthermore, all participants also discuss feeling stigmatized from their enrollment and how that caused problems with family members, or they choose not to disclose information about their enrollment again.

Combinations

Lastly, for social support, I will provide a few examples that include a combination of some of the four mentioned sub-themes. Participant 12, a Caucasian cisgender female with three dependents, provides an example with supportive and unsupportive family members:

> It differed on who it was, my parents were super supportive, Frank's parents were very embarrassed, almost like it was a stigma on them that we were enrolled (it reflected poorly on them). They did not want to help with the kids or anything and that we had made a bad decision, and because of that decision we had shamed them. We explained to them that it is temporary thing; we did not plan on staying on it forever. Frank was finishing up medical school and we get residency money so it was only for a two-year period in which we needed help with food money. It made us have a falling out with his parents, not just over the SNAP, but the reaction from us enrolling. I said well if it hurts you that we are enrolled, then you can help us get off of it. They were like no, you need to pull yourself up by your bootstraps; well, that is exactly what we are trying to do. (Personal communication, August 6, 2020)

Participant 12 is discussing that her family was supportive, but her husband's family was not. Several themes from iterative process are found in this example, including judgment/stigma, temporary enrollment, social support, embarrassment, and transitional state. Participant 12's response is a good example of how a participant can face different forms of support or the lack thereof while enrolled in SNAP.

Participant 5, a Hispanic cisgender male with four dependents, also notes having a vocal family member who does not support his SNAP enrollment, and his father who does support his enrollment:

> Always that fear, and in fact that more of a perceived completely hid it from my parents, especially my mom; I did not feel comfortable telling them with the exception from my father. Because I know that I would have been verbally abused by mother; she would not have been happy to know that I was on it, so I hid that in shame because of that. She has talked about it in the past that people that are on SNAP are lazy people who aren't working for their money. That it is a shameful thing to rely on an entity other than yourself to receive food, I know she would have done that to me. (Personal communication, July 6, 2020)

As with participant 12, participant 5 also feels judgment/stigma and embarrassment from enrollment because of a family member. Both of these examples highlight the struggle of receiving poor family support and having supportive family members, and the importance of having a supportive family.

While there are other examples of unsupportive family members and positive support, there are also examples of participants who have positive support from both friends and family members, such as participant 2, a Caucasian cisgender male with four dependents:

> YES, we would talk about my situation married with two kids, and having a hard time finding employment it was a little bit difficult. Talking to family about and to take advantage of the programs that are out there. So we applied, we talked about the amount that we were receiving; it was helpful for us and made it possible for us to survive instead of starving to death. We were pretty open to our family and friends because we were struggling so much. Family and friends were supportive but did not give us any money or anything. (Personal communication, July 18, 2020)

Unlike participants 12 and 5, participant 2 does not describe any judgment or embarrassment from his enrollment on SNAP, and though his family did not provide any tangible support, he states that it helped him through enrollment by allowing him to be open about their situation. Participant 18, a cisgender, Caucasian female with two dependents, had a similar experience while discussing the types of support received,

> All of them, tangible; my family did let us move back in their house with an extremely reduced rent, with the understanding that I would be paying for amenities now. The emotional came from the same place. Informational, my friends pointed me in the place to get some relief to build up again. (Personal communication, August 20, 2020)

Finally, participant 9 describes how she balances privacy and her enrollment on SNAP based on past negative experiences about her friends, but positive support from her mom:

> I have brought up with my mom and some friends. But mostly with people who have been enrolled in the past. Because they fully understand they know fully what this process entails. They understand the looks and how people look at you. Aside from that if they have never been on it they do not pay attention to what is around them. You look at it differently if you have been on it. (Personal communication, July 21, 2020)

I find all of these responses enlightening with how they are describing a process in which they share their enrollment but also the importance of having someone with whom to share the day-to-day information about enrollment, and how that process can help participants with the stigma. Overall, these examples provide for a unique analysis in terms of the benefits of social support and dealing with stigma. In research question 5.2, I analyzed if social support received from members of social circles during one's SNAP enrollment would positively or negatively impact enrollment, and I found that social support can do both.

SOCIAL SUPPORT AND SNAP ENROLLMENT IMPLICATIONS

While it is important to consider the stigmatizing experiences of an individual enrolled in SNAP and the possible ramifications, understanding how social support received from members of one's social circles impacts enrollment both negatively and positively is vital as well. Research Question 5.2 was formulated to answer the question of how social support received (if any) impacts enrollment on SNAP. As a reminder, 17 of the 19 participants reported receiving social support of some kind with 15 participants mentioning either supportive family or friends and 9 participants reporting unsupportive family or friends. Above in social support, I detailed the definitions of unsupportive/supportive friends and family but did not apply the types of social support to participants. In the 17 responses, there does not appear to be a cohesive theme across the different types of social support, tangible, emotional, and informational support, but a brief discussion of the type of social support and the 15 participants may provide some insight. In total, eight participants mentioned receiving tangible support (such as money, diapers, baby food, etc.), nine received emotional support (family or friends offering their support while the individual is enrolled in SNAP or providing a shoulder to vent on), and nine received informational support (help to enroll on the program itself, a person at the SNAP office, or a caseworker helping). Of the 17 responses, some participants received multiple types of support. Of the 15 responses with supportive family or friends, one individual said that tangible benefits helped the most while the person was enrolled on SNAP, six said informational support, and five said emotional support; some did not respond to the question about the most helpful support. Though not specifically asked in the interview, there seems to be an overall lack of esteem support, meaning that while families and friends may be overall supportive of enrolling on SNAP, they do not help build their self-esteem by suggesting that they have the skills and abilities to overcome. In fact, many responses indicated previously show that some responses by family members and friends can lower self-esteem, especially those that suggest "Why don't you go get another job," which then can lead to feelings of shame and failure. Because the numbers are not useful on their own, I went back to the interviews to determine if there was a difference between unsupportive/supportive family and friends to the type of social support reported as being received.

Nine participants reported having unsupportive family or friends, compared to 11 who had supportive friends and 15 had supportive family members. Many of these participants reported having both an unsupportive family member and a supportive family member. Participants who had unsupportive family members such as participants 1, 3, 5, 7, 8, 9, 11, and 12 also reported many of the other themes. For example, participant 1, an African American cisgender female, reported having no social support, avoiding discussion of her enrollment, actual verbal judgment from her enrollment, was worried about being considered lazy, and said that while SNAP is valuable, it encourages poverty and stigma from the lack of education and information. Because of participant 1's stigmatizing experiences, she chose to not disclose to others her enrollment, and in turn did not receive any social support. Similarly, participant 11, a Caucasian cisgender male, reported feeling embarrassed, actual verbal judgment, felt like a failure for needing to enroll, avoided discussion of SNAP, and received only minimal informational support from a local SNAP office. Because of his experiences, he chose to keep his enrollment from others and did not receive any social support from family or friends. Participant 9 also received very little social support and also experienced actual verbal and nonverbal judgment, felt embarrassed, hid card and enrollment, was asked to commit fraud, was accused of fraud, her children received social support from teachers, but she only received informational support to help be enrolled. Participant 9 was also emotional and cried during the interview process because she said she was frustrated that she could not share her experiences with others because of fear of judgment as seen in this comment,

> Yes, it does helps me to be able to express how it makes you feel. My voice is being heard in the project, though my name is written, it doesn't matter. I hope it gets others who have not been on it can see what others go through. It helps a lot to know that the feelings are out there. (Personal communication, July 21, 2020)

Participant 9 is highlighting how having her voice heard makes her feel better that her experiences may help another individual not have to experience the instances of judgment that she has received from her ex-husband in particular. Similarly, participant 10 reported having a supportive mom but unsupportive friends. She also reported actual verbal judgment, avoiding discussion of SNAP, and hiding her card. Furthermore, she indicated that she has received no social support even from her supportive mom. These four participants highlight the lack of social support for individuals who are enrolled in SNAP, unless that support comes from selected family and friends.

While participants 1, 9, 10, and 11 reported having very little social support from family and friends, participants 3, 5, 7, 8, 12, and 19 all reported having some positive social support from family but also nonsupport. Participant 3, a Caucasian cisgender female, reported that while her sister-in-law was unsupportive of her while she was enrolled on SNAP, all other family members were positive. Even though she reported having actual verbal judgment (from her sister-in-law), was accused of abuse, and had food choices judged, she still found SNAP enrollment to be valuable. She also reported that having informational support was essential to her enrollment and is the reason she continues to enroll. Participant 8 also found that informational support was very helpful to her while she was enrolled. Participant 8, a Caucasian cisgender female, reported having both supportive and unsupportive family and experienced embarrassment, actual verbal and nonverbal judgment, hid card and enrollment, avoided discussion about enrollment, and had food choices judged. She had also shared that even though she did not feel much stigma when she was first enrolled, the stigma came later. She said that she received no emotional support and received some tangible support from the state; she felt that informational support was the most valuable if a person would help her through it in the form of an agency. Lastly, participant 12 (Caucasian cisgender female) also had both unsupportive and supportive families. From having unsupportive family, she reports embarrassment, avoiding discussion, judged food choices, hiding card, and has received actual verbal and nonverbal judgment. She noted that she has received emotional support from a small group of people and that it has been very important to overcoming the stigma:

> Yeah, all three, tangible (my parents really helped for each bag of diapers I got, they got one, cribs, they were so excited for the babies that they wanted to help in any way). My parents were the ones who told me to enroll, and that is when I signed up online. Emotional support was a small group of people my parents and some close friends I shared our struggles with who had struggles themselves, so they understood what we were going through. I chose who I told the enrollment to. Emotional support—it just made it really instrumental to lifting the shame and just doing it. (Personal communication, August 6, 2020)

Even though she is emphasizing the importance of the social support that she has received, she still ends by describing how she chooses to control her disclosure of her enrollment. She is describing in detail how the CPM theory in chapter 3 can be applied to many of the SNAP participants' narratives; if there is some type of turbulence or impact to one's identity, a participant chooses to keep SNAP enrollment private. Overall, the individuals who reported having unsupportive family members either received very little support or primarily were given informational or some emotional support. Participants who had unsupportive family and friends highlight the need of having positive and constructive social support while enrolled on SNAP to help manage the stigma from being enrolled.

Unlike participants who had unsupportive family members and friends, those who had supportive family and friends reported less judgment and reported SNAP as more valuable compared to those who had unsupportive family members. For example, participant 6, a Hispanic cisgender male, reported having no judgment or stigma, and received emotional and informational support from both family and friends. Participant 14 also reported having supportive family and friends and reported no judgment or stigma and received emotional, tangible, and informational support from her social circles. Not all participants who reported supportive family and friends reported having received verbal judgment such as participants 13 and 18, but they both had supportive family and friends who provided emotional and informational support. Having both supportive family and friends led to reporting more received social support, regardless of the type of support, and having more individuals one could talk to about SNAP was important. For example, when participant 9 mentions that she has only discussed with her mom and friends who are currently enrolled, she is referring to having a shared past history of discussion of SNAP and believes that if she shares this information, she anticipates a more positive reaction from those particular individuals. Having a positive prior history of discussion and anticipated response talk encouraged her disclosure to those individuals about her stigmatizing experiences. The same cannot be said for participant 1 who describes how she had shared with her parents one time about her SNAP enrollment but was berated for enrolling. She then chose to not further disclose her SNAP enrollment to others resulting in very little social support while she was enrolled. In terms of the chain of discourses, participant 1's parents' assumption of the cultural view of SNAP, the negative history of discussion and assumed negative anticipated response caused her to not share further. The rich dynamics between supportive family and friends lend further support that the chain of discourses and RDT also play a key role in support.

Overall, the primary difference between participants who had supportive family and friends and those who did not was the lack of or less social support than those with stronger social support systems. Individuals who had unsupportive family or friends also reported more judgment, feelings of failure, fear of being seen as lazy, and embarrassed when compared to those that had support, which relates to the earlier discussion of the lack of or negative esteem support given to these individuals. They also reported having little to no social support received, whereas those who reported having supportive family and friends never reported receiving no social support. Interestingly, if an individual had a supportive and unsupportive member of his or her social circles, the person reported some judgment and was more likely to still need to avoid discussion of SNAP enrollment. Individuals who reported only supportive family and friends did not report judgment or a fear of disclosing their enrollment. The differences between supportive and unsupportive family and friends highlight a great need for positive social support for individuals while they are enrolled on SNAP to help them cope with some of the stigmas they are receiving.

CONCLUSION

Interview findings indicate support for the statistical findings, suggesting that people on SNAP experience feelings of stigma by reporting themes of embarrassment, judgment, failure, and laziness. Furthermore, SNAP participants also have fears of disclosing their SNAP enrollment (based on prior or anticipated experiences) to individuals who may further judge them so they choose to not disclose their enrollment, avoid discussion of the topic, or hide their card or enrollment from others in the grocery store. Though fewer in number than total stigma and concern for disclosing SNAP enrollment to a specific person, participants still reported stigma that impacted their identity as seen in anticipated consequences from disclosing SNAP enrollment stigma. However, the interviews add to the discussion of stigma to important findings regarding social support. The more supportive members of one's social circles there are, the less reported judgment, and more received support was reported. Individuals who had unsupportive family or friends also reported receiving none to very little support and experiencing many of the found themes. The findings from the interviews also help to align the statistical data into personal actual experiences of everyday SNAP enrollment and help provide a foundation in which theory can be applied to explain many of the behaviors found in both the surveys and interviews, which is discussed in chapter 3.

In chapter 9, I will further discuss these implications about the negative effects of stigma and the positive impacts of social support in the light of two themes that were found to be factors that also influenced enrollment—race and political ideology.

Chapter 9

Factors That Influence Enrollment and Implications from Findings

Throughout this book, I have described a variety of factors that were found to significantly impact enrollment on SNAP, including stigma in chapter 6, disclosure concerns in chapter 7, and social support in chapter 8. Throughout these chapters, I have included a discussion about the social determinants of health and how the view of stigma, disclosure concerns, and social support can differ based on a multitude of factors. I will provide a brief discussion about the findings for the social determinants of health and SNAP enrollment.

SOCIAL DETERMINANTS OF HEALTH AND ENROLLMENT

In chapters 1 and 2, I discussed how the social determinants of health could be used as a possible framework to analyze how certain demographic variables are present in individuals who face daily hardships in poverty. The social determinants analyzed in my study are migrant status, immigrant status, race, and educational attainment. To determine how these determinants (the independent variables) impact individuals who are currently and no longer enrolled in SNAP (dependent variable), a logistic regression was used. The logistic regression for the social determinants of health (demographic variables) was significant (Wald χ^2 (8) = 30.14, p = 0.000). Please note that these results do not include any of the variables relating to stigma, only the social determinants of health (demographic variables).

According to the results from the logistic regression, only migrant status and immigrant status have a significant difference for individuals enrolled and no longer enrolled. To explain the differences in effects size, I have included both the odds ratio and predicted probabilities. Note the coefficient should be interpreted as a one-unit change in the independent variable (IV) results in the specific coefficient change in the log-odds ratio that the dependent variable (DV) is 1. For example, for migrant status for every one-unit change, there is 0.38 increase in the log-odds ratio that an individual is currently enrolled. Similarly, for immigrant status, for every one-unit change, there is 0.81 increase in the log-odds ratio that an individual is currently enrolled. The differences in the odds ratio for immigrant and migrant status indicate a larger effect for immigrant status on current enrollment. To help better explain the effect size of the logistic regression coefficients, the minimum predicted probability for migrant status is 0.73 with a maximum of 0.98 for a change of 0.25, whereas, immigrant status has a minimum predicted probability of 0.70 and a maximum of 0.96 with a change of 0.26.

Immigrant status had a slightly higher impact on current enrollment than migrant status. The results indicate that as an individual has more members of the household who have a migrant or temporary worker status, the individual has a higher probability of being enrolled in SNAP than individuals who are not migrant or temporary workers. Similarly, as an individual reports being an immigrant or has family members who are immigrants, the person has a higher probability of being currently enrolled in SNAP than individuals who reported otherwise. However, please note that even for individuals who did not select being a migrant or temporary worker (the minimum) or a first-generation immigrant (the minimum), the probability of being enrolled was still high (70% or higher), but the difference among the groups is significant.

Throughout the chapters, migrant status and immigrant status are continuously found to be factors that influence enrollment on SNAP, both in the statistical data and the interview data. In fact, all statistical models have migrant and immigrant status as significant factors not only for enrollment but for all of the stigma variables as well. Migrant/temporary workers and first-generation immigrants continuously reported having more total stigma and concerns for disclosing their SNAP enrollment. Though there could be many factors such as migrant and temporary workers are more likely to live in poverty (Wolfe et al., 2020) or that first-generation immigrants have not yet attained the "American Dream," they are beyond the scope of this project but deserve further study about SNAP enrollment to improve their overall experiences while they are enrolled. None of their specific responses indicated a cohesive list, but many immigrant and migrant temporary workers mentioned that the cultural elements of SNAP are more salient (whether this is from the general political environment in the USA is unclear). In addition to migrant/temporary workers and first-generation immigrants, later statistical models that controlled for continued enrollment and other factors also indicated that the number of members in the household, education attainment, generation of SNAP enrollment, and gender significantly differed for enrollment and stigma. In the interview data, the theme of race came up several times but was not statistically significant.

RACE

Seven participants either mentioned the race of individuals who had verbally judged them or the participants mentioned the stigma received because of their own race. Though the statistical findings did not support a racial difference in SNAP enrollment, the responses from the interviews may help clarify. Participant 2, a Caucasian male, mentioned on the Internet the race of an individual using SNAP benefits,

> The issue I have with the program overall is that it does not limit you on what you buy, such as blue crab that I saw on a YouTube video where an African-American woman used food stamps to purchase the crabs. I wish that I was able to eat blue crab when I was getting them. (Personal communication, July 20, 2020)

Here participant 2 is not only discussing the race of the participant using her SNAP benefits but also judging the choice of food the person has received.

Participant 13, an African American cisgender female, also discusses the race of SNAP recipients at her previous employment:

> I remember when I would manage Office Depot, food stamps have been stigmatized for black people and not white people. When people would pay, you would see what was in their wallet, and it would be people that you could tell, people that you would not assume that have food stamp cards. It would be people who you would not think. One white man tried to convince me that it was a debit/credit card that I saw because he was ashamed. They appeared as well dressed and put to do, you know they appeared that way. It was funny cause customers would say, "Well, it is primarily black people who are enrolled." Do you know how many well-to-do white people are living with SNAP? (Personal communication, July 27, 2020)

Participant 13 discusses not only the race of an individual that attempted to hide the SNAP card but also the stigma that she feels she is experiencing because of herself being a black woman.

Similarly, participant 9, a Caucasian, cisgender female, mentions how she feels that she receives stigma because of her race:

> You know my mom is of Portuguese descent so she looks like the tiny Spanish lady because remember she looks nothing like me. That is a whole different

stigma than I do because I look white. They look at me like I am a white woman, you should be well taken care of; there's no reason whatsoever. It happens at work, too, all of the time because my maiden name and married name look Hispanic but I do not even though I am. (Personal communication, July 21, 2020)

Another example of a participant mentioning specifically the race of someone that makes them feel more stigmatized is from participant 5, a Hispanic, cisgender male:

That it is a shameful thing to rely on an entity other than yourself to receive food; I know she (mother) would have done that to me. Being from an Hispanic culture, a lot of Hispanics that are on it or at least the stigma that they are on it. A lot of pride specifically from her side of the family as poor as they were, they never considered help from the government that wasn't earned. (Personal communication, July 6, 2020)

Participant 5 is noting that he feels more stigmatized for his SNAP enrollment because his family is Hispanic, and he did not want to disappoint them. His description differs from participants 2, 13, and 9 because they are highlighting either themselves or individuals that they have felt stigmatized elsewhere.

Overall, there are several other examples that highlight the race of an individual in the grocery store as in participant 12, a Caucasian, cisgender female, "A white lady behind me said 'Oh look! Another one using the government'" (personal communication, August 6, 2020) or participant 13, an African American cisgender female:

You can look at people, this is a judgment, you can look at who is ringing people up at the registers and choose who I think will be less judgmental. And I will be honest and this is racist, if I see an older white lady, I will not go to her. Now, if it is younger white person, I may go to them because they do not know enough some of them, even some older black people. (Personal communication, July 27, 2020)

These examples and others indicate that one possible reason why race is not a statistically significant factor, such as different races see themselves as stigmatized more from their enrollment because of their race. The reported stigma is hard to determine who may feel more stigmatized on SNAP because of their race, but regardless, the responses indicate that race is an important factor in stigma and SNAP enrollment rather than one's own race or the race of others in the grocery store.

One last factor that may influence enrollment on SNAP, political ideology, was measured for in the statistical analysis but was found in the interview data.

POLITICAL IDEOLOGY

The last theme that I found was individuals indicating people's political ideology in their interviews. Please note that participants were not prompted to reveal their political ideology or political party affiliation, but these responses still came up in three participants' interviews. For example, participant 5, when asked who is concerned about receiving stigma from SNAP, he responds,

> My coworkers probably would not care. The people I work with are not in the same state, and one is very liberal so he probably would support it . . . He (father) is very conservative, but also very pragmatic, even he didn't agree, it did not matter. I would visit and they would give me $300. (Personal communication, July 20, 2020)

While participant 5 specifically mentions political ideology of his coworkers and his father, participant 12 mentions ideology in a discussion about received stigma (specifically about food choices) and losing family members because of their enrollment:

> Family members, this did happen, they did distance themselves from me after making some ugly comments to us. I have some first cousins that are very conservative; they were going off on poor people using their tax dollars on lobster and steak fillets, so I had to say something, "Listen to me, I am on SNAP; we cannot afford lobster. If I do buy lobster it is my budget for the next 3 weeks. It is unfeasible for that, I was like you are wrong." They were shocked and said, Oh so you are on SNAP, and I said yeah because Frank and I are in college, and we need it. Then they said well maybe you should not have had kids. (Personal communication, August 11, 2020)

A similar use of ideology can be found in participant 19's (Caucasian, cisgender female) examples of stigmatizing experiences that she has had when she was enrolled on SNAP:

> The only person outside of the broader societal and internal dialogue was one close relative who made some hateful insinuations about work ethic, which is really ironic because at the time, I was working 3 part-time jobs, and this

relative made some insinuations about using up taxpayers' money and taking it away from other people. One of those typical offensive conservative lines #comebackwhenyoucontribute, as if paying taxes is the only way to contribute, as if you do not pay taxes when you are on SNAP, even though we did. So many things that were offensive. (Personal communication, August 28, 2020).

Overall, the idea that participants responded about political ideology without being prompted made the theme a very interesting finding that warrants further research.

Throughout my analysis, so many factors have been found to influence enrollment on SNAP, and still, one new theme emerged from the interview data indicating there are so many possible factors that can influence enrollment. In the social ecological model in chapter 2, I discussed how elements like race, stigma, social support, migrant status, immigrant status, and education attainment can impact individuals across different levels of the self, and may in turn impact across life spans as indicated in some responses. Furthermore, participants who had multiple social determinants of health, specifically migrant and temporary workers and first-generation immigrants, reported more stigma from enrollment. There are further details about these differences in chapters 6, 7, and 8. These differences also impacted disclosure of SNAP enrollment as seen in chapter 3 in which I discussed how a multitude of factors can impact relationships such as history of discussion, cultural components and anticipated response talk in RDT and the chain of discourses, and the privacy turbulence found in CPM. Overall, this study scratches the surface of the many factors and the complex nature of stigma and social support impacting participants who are enrolled on SNAP.

IMPLICATIONS OF THE STUDY

The explanatory sequential mixed-methods designed study allowed for a richer understanding of stigma and social support and SNAP enrollment than would have occurred with a simpler design. The surveys provided the specific elements of stigma that significantly impact SNAP enrollment—total stigma (Herek et al. stigma scale), anticipated consequences from disclosing SNAP enrollment stigma (DISC-12), concern for disclosing SNAP enrollment to a specific person stigma (Wright et al. stigma scale), and past consequences for disclosing SNAP enrollment stigma (DISC-12). The survey data also identified the specific demographic variables, that are also social determinants of health, that more strongly impacted the experience of being enrolled in SNAP, specifically migrant status, immigrant status, members of the household, higher educational attainment, and generation of SNAP enrollment. Most of the statistical findings from are supported in the interviews; SNAP participants do report judgment and total stigma from being enrolled, disclosure concerns are present, and fewer participants reported anticipating consequences from disclosing SNAP enrollment stigma than those who reported total stigma. However, the interview results are harder to determine if there is much of a difference in the number of reported stigma variables and the impact on current and past recipients. Though it is harder to determine a difference in current and past members, I have reported differences in the narratives for individuals who had been enrolled, were unenrolled, and then because of the COVID pandemic, they had to re-enroll. One difference between the interview data and the survey results, is the lack of support for the past consequences from disclosing SNAP enrollment stigma concern variable in the surveys that related to losing family members or friends due to their enrollment. Only one individual mentioned having lost family members because of enrollment, and one other said he or she may have lost friends on Facebook because of the posts about SNAP support, but the person was unclear if that had actually happened. Many of the responses indicated that while there are consequences from disclosing their SNAP enrollment to others, it rarely ends in a complete disconnection from those specific friends and family, which overall is a good thing because results indicate that positive social support from friends and family leads to less feelings of judgment, embarrassment, feelings of laziness, feelings of failure, and so on.

However, these were the only two factors that were not found as clearly in the interviews as they are in the survey data. Interview findings support the statistical findings that migrant workers, immigrants, higher education attainment individuals, generation SNAP, and larger households do experience more stigma but are more likely to be enrolled at some point because, even with the COVID-19 pandemic, I was able to recruit several of these individuals and many had intersectionality of all variables. Furthermore, both studies do show that individuals who are enrolled on SNAP do experience many levels of stigma at one time, and when individuals in their support circles are not supportive, they feel worse about their enrollment. These individuals are already some of the most vulnerable populations. This situation is very troubling considering that SNAP is supposed to help individuals already living in extreme poverty by providing support to help feed themselves and their families. Finding again in the surveys and interviews that individuals feel they are stigmatized for their enrollment because of the cultural assumptions of the program is terrible. While total stigma and judgment are bad enough, some individuals did feel that their enrollment is at war with their identity, and they feel worse about themselves for having to be enrolled. While stigma can be seen as a negative consequence from SNAP enrollment, the presence of social support in the interviews highlights that support can help alleviate some of the negative attributes from SNAP. More participants reported positive support from family members and friends than those who reported negative support or no support, but those that did report negative or no support faced more negative ramifications from enrollment than those with only positive support, suggesting that individuals enrolled in SNAP need to be provided positive support from family and friends. A quick Facebook search indicated that while there are SNAP support groups, they are primarily used to share information about SNAP, not how to deal with the stigma and discrimination from enrollment, suggesting that these types of groups are not enough to deal with the stigma from enrollment, especially if they are one of the few individuals who reported not having any social support while they were enrolled on SNAP. Future campaigns and interventions could be to form SNAP social support groups to help fill the gaps or address the negative support present in SNAP participants' lives. Furthermore, though not explicitly studied, stigma and discrimination and the variables that are social determinants of health can negatively impact one's health. Thus, it is important to determine some methods that can help improve SNAP enrollment. Some individuals highlighted that there are ways in which the program could be amended to help with this stigma, like better education, more transparency with fraud, and less rigid cutoffs of the program. However, these changes are beyond the scope of this book, but more campaigns or interventions may be needed to help those individuals that feel stigmatized while they are enrolled. Many of the complaints found in the study could be alleviated or lessened by policy improvement on the program and providing of services, such as a system that still provides some amount of SNAP allotment for individuals who no longer reach the cutoff amount (make too much money) or stronger support groups available for individuals who feel the most stigma from enrollment. The study highlights that while the program has many positive attributes, there is still much that can be done to help populations in need. (Limitations from the study can be found in appendix F.)

FUTURE RESEARCH

Future research into the SNAP program needs to be performed to include the voices of individuals that are often marginalized and stigmatized. I would suggest trying to recruit more individuals who are immigrants and migrant and temporary workers and analyzing their experiences on SNAP. Because these individuals consistently in the surveys reported that they felt more stigmatized, and while I was able to recruit some for the interviews, this was particularly difficult because of COVID. I would also suggest performing similar studies on other welfare assistance programs such as WIC (which was mentioned several times in the interview data), temporary assistance for needy families (TANF), Medicaid, supplemental security income (SSI), and so on. Many of these programs also serve communities that are under-researched and could be under similar circumstances as those that are enrolled on SNAP but may face different stigma and varying levels of social support. Furthermore, the other welfare programs may have more or less stigma than others, in which participants of the different programs may psychologically distance themselves from other members of the same welfare programs. Some participants in the interviews reported negative views of SNAP participants, even though they were also SNAP participants suggesting that SNAP participants may distance themselves from other SNAP users, indicating that further research is needed to address why this type of disclosure happens. Lastly, I also suggest further campaigns, case studies, and preventions to help improve individuals in different states to have better social support teams to help with individuals especially in the time of COVID in which many are in need of social support as more individuals have had to enroll on SNAP because of job loss. I would also like to research more into applying the SMC to SNAP participants, CPM to disclosure of SNAP enrollment, as well as RDT to help further illuminate the impacts of relationships while enrolled on SNAP, specifically in significant others. These suggestions are by no means a conclusive list of areas of future research but a few different areas into which research could broaden.

CONCLUSION

Through the use of the explanatory sequential mixed-methods design of the current study, useful insight into the daily experiences of stigma and social support and SNAP enrollment was found. The statistical portion of the study helped narrow down many of the different types of possible SNAP stigma to four main variables. Of the four main variables, only consequences stigma was not found in the interviews. Having a manageable number of stigma variables helped to provide a more concise and usable list of questions for the interview process. The interview process provided additional data to the survey data which already indicated that enrollment on SNAP was complicated and more complex than I had first believed. SNAP individuals face a number of different factors daily because of their SNAP enrollment, including stigma and judgment, but social support is a key element for individuals while they are enrolled. Having an individual or individuals who can provide any type of support is helpful, even if just to have an ear to listen.

While not everything about SNAP is reported to be damaging, as participants did say that it was a valuable program, there was an overarching idea that the program is not enough to help poverty and changes are needed, because even after many years, a large number of the individuals no longer enrolled could recall feelings of embarrassment, shame, and failure about their SNAP enrollment. Additionally, judgmental family or friends and the societal stigma of SNAP as a whole can have lifelong impacts on one's identity. The societal shame is further complicated when individuals have multiple levels of stigma, intersectionality, such as being an immigrant, a migrant or temporary worker, and multigenerational SNAP user all at one time. The damaging effects of stigma were less likely if participants had stronger and more supportive social circles. Individuals with more support reported less judgment than those who had less support, suggesting that more support groups are needed for participants of welfare assistance programs such as SNAP beyond simple information about the program in general. Many individuals who are enrolled in SNAP are already facing stigmatizing situations such as being impoverished, different racial and ethnic background, having higher educational attainment but not employment, and so on, before even applying, and this study provides a snapshot of the enrollment of SNAP and the many complex levels of stigma and judgment these individuals face daily.

Due to the lack of research on SNAP, the current study allows for further research into individuals who need the support but face obstacles because of their enrollment. Applying the data to the many theories has allowed for a more defined picture of the mechanics of disclosure of SNAP enrollment, the negative impacts of stigma on disclosure, and the importance of family and friend support. While the study provides but a small lens into a large complex world of SNAP enrollment, the results found paint a rich and unique perspective into a program that is often not researched. The results provide more information beyond whether SNAP is a healthy recourse for individuals, the specific dietary functions of the food consumed on SNAP, and the fact that people do feel stigmatized on SNAP. The study adds that there are many different elements of stigma that can influence current participants more than past recipients, and that past recipients can still feel stigma from their enrollment after many years. Additionally, the study shows that these different levels of stigma can also be influenced by the lack or inclusion of social support.

To my knowledge and research, no study has applied the RDT and the chain of discourses or the CPM theory to SNAP enrollment. Both theories highlight how the decisions to disclose enrollment and to discuss stigma are based and grounded in communication and relationships. The data found adds to the very limited amount of research in SNAP by providing specific experiences and internal mechanisms of dealing with the stigma from SNAP enrollment and disclosing that enrollment to others. Hopefully applying these results on a larger scale will help improve the lives of individuals living on welfare assistance in the future to provide a healthier lifestyle for themselves and their family members.

Appendix A

Factor Analysis

A separate principal component factor analysis was performed using an orthogonal varimax rotation for all three instruments—the Herek et al. stigma scale, the DISC-12, and the Wright et al. disclosure concerns scale. All rules for the orthogonal varimax rotation factor analysis are described in Hair et al. (2009).

HEREK ET AL.'S STIGMA SCALE

The Herek et al.'s scale consists of items from enacted, perceived, vicarious, felt normative, and internalized stigma for a total of five variables. The initial eigenvalues indicated that only three factors scored above a 1: factor 1 (eigenvalue = 9.33) which explained 54% of the variance, factor 2 (eigenvalue = 1.18) explained 7% of the variance, and factor 3 (eigenvalue = 1.11) explained 7% of the variance. Several items were cross loaded on multiple factors with less than 0.20 difference after the orthogonal varimax rotation was used and were subsequently removed. Thus, the factors needed further examination as recommended by Hair et al. (2009).

The first item removed was perceived 1, "People view me differently because of my enrollment in SNAP," because it loaded 0.48 on factor 1 and 0.54 on factor 2 with a 0.06 difference between factors. The next item that needed to be removed was felt 2, "People in my state disapprove of SNAP use," with a cross loading on factor 2 (0.52) and factor 3 (0.44). Next, vicarious 4, "Other people I know have had bad experiences with other customers at the store over SNAP," was removed because it loaded 0.62 on factor 1 and 0.52 on factor 3 with a 0.09 difference. The fourth item eliminated was perceived 3, "People view me differently at checkout in a store because of my SNAP enrollment," because the item loaded on both factor 1 (0.55) and factor 2 (0.42) for a difference of 0.13.

Next, the following rotation indicated that vicarious 2, "I know close friends who have been mistreated because of their enrollment on SNAP," needed to be removed because of cross loadings on factor 1 (0.64) and factor 3 (0.52). After eliminating vicarious 2, the eigenvalues indicated two factors and dropped the third. The sixth item eliminated was internal 3, "I feel embarrassed for my enrollment on SNAP," because it cross loaded by less than 0.01 on factor 1 (0.52) and factor 2 (0.53). Felt 1, "People in my local community (your town) disapprove of SNAP use," cross loaded on factor 1 (0.51) and factor 2 (0.62) and was eliminated. Lastly, the final item, perceived 2, "I see negative comments about SNAP users on social media and think that the messages are directed at me," was removed for cross loading on factors 1 (0.64) and 2 (0.49).

After eliminating these identified items that cross loaded on multiple factors, a new analysis resulted in only one factor with an eigenvalue of 5.08 and explaining 57% of the variance remained. The remaining items that did not cross load on any other factor after the orthogonal rotation are enacted 1 (0.83), enacted 2 (0.85), enacted 3 (0.79), enacted 4 (0.84), vicarious 1 (0.48), vicarious 3 (0.76), felt 3 (0.62), internal 1 (0.72), and internal 2 (0.80). All of these items include elements of physical impacts from stigma such as shame, name-calling, mistreatment, or disapproval suggesting that participants viewed SNAP enrollment as an overall stigmatizing situation and interpreted the questions about stigma similarly rather than different distinct dimensions. Because of the combined elements of all the different types of stigma factor 1, the Herek's stigma variables will now all be called "total stigma." This could be an example of applying an instrument that has been typically used in HIV/AIDS studies to SNAP enrollment and not be interpreted as separate and unique dimensions of stigma as those participants did. No collinearity was found among the items on the scale. Lastly, the Cronbach α for the nine items that make up stigma is 0.90.

DISC-12

A separate factor analysis was generated for the DISC-12. The DISC-12 consists of items about the sources of stigma received including from family members, friends, work, and socioeconomic status (SES). The initial eigenvalues indicated two specific factors: factor 1 with a score of 7.32 explaining 66% of the variance and factor 2 with an eigenvalue of 1.04, explaining 9% of the variance. In the initial factor analysis, several items indicated cross loading on both factors. The first variable to be removed for cross loading was family 1, "I feel the need to hide my enrollment on SNAP from my family," with a score of 0.65 on factor 1 and 0.54 on factor 2 with a 0.11 difference. Next, family 2, "I fear a negative reaction from family if I discuss my enrollment in SNAP," was eliminated for cross loading on factor 1 (0.67) and factor 2 (0.49) with a difference of 0.18. No other items were eliminated. Friends 1 and friends 2 were not removed from the factor analysis even though they both had a 0.40 loading on factor 1 but a high loading on factor 2. According to Hair et al. (2009), the difference must be greater than 0.20 to keep in the model; for friends 1, the difference is 0.35 and 0.36 for friends 2. Removing these will cause the loadings to all be on factor 1 and could possibly skew the data.

After all cross-loaded items were removed, five items loaded with factor 1: Family 3, "I have lost family members because of my enrollment on SNAP"; family 4, "Because of my enrollment on SNAP, family members communicate less with me"; friends 3, "I have lost close friends because of my enrollment on SNAP"; friends 4, "Because of my enrollment on SNAP close friends communicate less with me"; and work 3, "Because of my enrollment on SNAP, the people I work with (coworkers, boss, associates, customers, etc.) communicate less with me." The items that load on factor 1 suggest that as individuals disclose their SNAP status to others, they experience stigma and discrimination that leads to more physical losses in one's social circles such as family members, friends, and coworkers. For this implied reason, I suggest labeling this factor, "Past consequences from disclosing SNAP enrollment." The Cronbach α for past consequences from disclosing SNAP enrollment is 0.93.

Factor 2 includes friends 1, "I feel the need to hide my enrollment on SNAP from my friends," friends 2, "I fear a negative reaction from friends if I discuss my enrollment in SNAP," work 1 "I feel the need to hide my enrollment on SNAP from the people I work with (coworkers, boss, associates, customers, etc.)," and work 2, "I fear a negative reaction from the people I work with (coworkers, boss, associates, customers, etc.) when I discuss my enrollment in SNAP." Unlike factor 1, the assumption is not that the individuals have disclosed their SNAP enrollment to others, but they fear how others would respond if they knew about their enrollment. Factor 2 indicates the fear or worry to disclose the enrollment to friends and coworkers. These opinions could be formed from hearing about others' experiences with SNAP such as vicarious stigma, previous experience with disclosing to others, or from the concern of how any received stigma could negatively influence one's personal identity. Thus, I will be labeling this factor "Anticipated consequences from disclosing SNAP enrollment stigma." The variance for factor 1 is 3.87 (explaining 43%) and 3.04 (explaining 34%) for factor 2. The Cronbach α for anticipated consequences from disclosing SNAP enrollment stigma is 0.88.

Lastly of the DISC-12 variables, total SES stigma behaves very differently from its other variables and loads on a singular factor; no aspects of total SES cross loaded. The Cronbach α for total SES stigma is 0.83.

WRIGHT ET AL. DISCLOSURE CONCERNS

A third and final principal component factor analysis with orthogonal/varimax rotation was used for the Wright et al. disclosure concern instrument. A total of nine items are included in the instruments. The nine items are loaded on two factors. The eigenvalue for factor 1 is 4.66, explaining 51% of the variance, and 1.36 for factor 2 with 15% of the variance. After the Varimax rotation, factor 1 has a variance score of 3.64 and factor 2 has 2.37. No items cross loaded on both factors. Factor 1 or "Concern for disclosing SNAP enrollment to a specific person" includes the items that relate to whom one is concerned with disclosing SNAP enrollment: "disclose close friends" (0.83), "disclose friends" (0.83), "disclose parents or guardians" (0.78), "disclose significant other" (0.80), "disclose work relationships" (0.70), and "disclose stranger" (0.66). Note the "disclose to close family members" such as brothers and sisters was dropped from the analysis because it was found that this item had over 40 missing data points. The Cronbach α for "concern for disclosing SNAP enrollment to a specific person" is 0.89, while factor 2 or total disclosure concern consists of disclosure 1 (0.79), disclosure 2 (0.83), and disclosure 3 (0.83). The Cronbach α for generalized SNAP enrollment disclosure concern is 0.80.

Appendix B
Past and Present Methodology

PRIOR PILOT STUDIES

Through the course of several pilot studies, I have narrowed down the variables that may impact enrollment on SNAP. Furthermore, I have also improved my data collection methods based on the shortfalls of the prior studies. Over the course of four pilot studies involving SNAP, WIC, stigma, and social support, I have decided on the following measures to help answer the primary question of how stigma and social support impact enrollment on SNAP.

Pilot Study 1

The first study analyzed both WIC and SNAP participants in a sociology course. I analyzed stigma, and social ties broadly using the DISC-12 instrument and the RAND social battery (along with other variables that do not pertain to this dissertation). Participants were recruited from Amazon's MTurk with a total sample of 254 individuals. Of those participants, 128 were currently enrolled in SNAP or WIC and 126 were no longer enrolled. Results indicated no support for differences in experienced stigma across WIC and SNAP participants but for differences across minority groups. Second, no support was found for WIC and SNAP enrollment and the number of social ties. When analyzing the results from this study, I realized there were several factors that were not being considered. Although DISC does provide an analysis of the sources of stigma, no questions address what type of stigma was experienced. To test the validity of both instruments at predicting stigma from welfare enrollment, I performed a second study that focused solely on the DISC-12 and RAND social health battery.

Pilot Study 2

The second study analyzed both the sources of stigma and some differences in social support across WIC and SNAP participants using the DISC-12 and RAND instruments. A total of 225 participants were recruited from local individuals enrolled in SNAP and Amazon's MTurk. No significant differences were found between WIC and SNAP participants for the number of family ties or friends ties. The only significant finding relating to social ties was that WIC participants met more with others than SNAP recipients. From the lack of significant findings concerning the RAND social health battery across both groups, I decided to longer use the instrument. The finding that WIC participants met more with others than SNAP participants led me to focus primarily on SNAP participants to determine why this was the case. While the finding that differences do exist across welfare programs was impactful, some of the quantitative findings for social support were not as useful and were difficult to understand, particularly the helpfulness of the support and the different types of support received. These findings suggested that a more interpretive approach might be more productive in teasing out how these different sources of support were perceived by the recipients of that support. In addition to findings for social support, results from the DISC-12 and measuring stigma were found. SNAP recipients reported having more stigma than WIC participants (t = 3.45, β = 0.38), whereas individuals who were enrolled in both experienced more stigma than either WIC or SNAP alone. Although the results indicating significance for stigma and SNAP enrollment have been important in shaping my current research, as with study 1, I felt that I needed to determine how the different types of stigma also influence enrollment.

Pilot Study 3

From these first two studies, I felt that the studies were too broad with smaller sample sizes which did not provide meaningful results that could be used to improve elements of SNAP for individuals enrolled. Through research, I came across Herek's different types of AIDS stigma and wanted to test to see if they were applicable to SNAP participants' experiences. A total of 102 participants were recruited using Amazon's MTurk engine and Louisiana State University's research participation system. I used the Generalized Structural Equation Modeling (GSEM) as a mean of analyzing the data. The likelihood to stay enrolled for longer on SNAP had several significant variables or close to significance (<0.10) including, the number of members of the household (positively), felt normative stigma (negatively more felt normative less likely to enroll), total internalized stigma (positively, the longer on SNAP, the more internalized stigma), and minority differences (individuals of African American descent had longer enrolled on SNAP compared to individuals of Asian descent). Next, based on a pairwise correlation, I included several interactions in the GSEM (denoted by the *) that were significant including education*enacted (the higher the education, the higher enacted stigma reported), migrant*vicarious stigma (negative, migrants that had more vicarious stigma were less likely to enroll), education*vicarious stigma (negative, similar as for migrants), education*felt normative (positive, more education, more felt normative stigma), family stigma *migrant (more family stigma for migrants, more likely to enroll longer), and friends stigma* migrant (more friends stigma for migrants, less likely to enroll). Results from the interactions suggest that while the variables alone may not significantly impact uniformly across individuals, they will differ per an individual's background. Through these significant results, I decided to include both DISC-12 and Herek's stigma to analyze the potential differences in experienced stigma and enrollment on SNAP.

Pilot Study 4

Over the course of the three pilot studies, I found an AIDS stigma instrument by Berger et al. (2001) which analyzed negative self-image, disclosure concerns, and concern for public attitudes. Berger's instrument inspired me because of the more communicative elements present in the instrument. The Berger instrument was the first instrument that I found that included disclosure concerns as a potential stigmatizing event. I wanted to determine if the instrument could be applied to SNAP participants. To do so, I recruited 148 participants from Amazon's MTurk Engine and Louisiana State University research participation system. In this pilot study, negative self-image and disclosure concerns were the only significant factors, with disclosure concerns having the most important finding. Individuals who experienced higher disclosure concerns about their enrollment on SNAP were less likely to continue their enrollment. That is, the longer a person was enrolled on SNAP, the lower their self-image. Once I began thinking about the impacts of lower self-image, I decided to remove the variable because it appears to conceptually overlap with perceived and internalized stigma. From the final pilot study, I found, in my opinion, one of the most important variables that could impact SNAP enrollment.

Thus, the instruments provided in this appendix were created over several projects and years to ensure that what I was trying to measure was indeed being measured to further provide assistance to individuals who need help the most.

Appendix B

CURRENT METHODOLOGY

To determine how stigma and social support impact enrollment on SNAP, I propose an explanatory sequential mixed-methods design study, first with a survey to determine what variables impact stigma and second an interview process that analyzes the differences in how received stigma is discussed via social support. An explanatory sequential mixed-methods design study is defined as,

> One in which the researcher first conducts quantitative research, analyzes the results, and then builds on the results to explain them in more detail with qualitative research. It is considered explanatory because the initial quantitative data results are explained further with the qualitative data. (Creswell & Creswell, 2018, p. 15)

The explanatory sequential mixed-methods design was selected to help narrow down the broad topic that is stigma to be able to ask more specific questions to SNAP participants, instead of prompting questions about general stigma. Prior studies have found that people feel stigmatized about their SNAP enrollment (Smith, 2007; Vancil, 2008; Fricke et al., 2015), but very little specific information about stigma is discussed. Thus, I wanted to analyze more specific elements of stigma but did not have a firm understanding of what stigma elements would be present, so a survey was needed first to determine what specific elements of stigma significantly impact enrollment. The explanatory design will help provide more context to an already complex topic, SNAP welfare stigma, into more useable information. Lastly, the explanatory nature will also allow for better-explained connections between the quantitative data about stigma and the social support responses found in the interview data.

Now that I have explained why I have chosen to use an explanatory sequential mixed-methods design, I will describe how participants were selected for the study. To be accepted for either study, participants must be either a current member or past member of SNAP regardless of time. First, enrollment on SNAP will be operationalized by analyzing the enrollment status of a participant, specifically if they are currently enrolled or enrolled in the past. Analyzing the enrollment status of a participant will provide insight into the differences that may be present across enrollees. Brown and Kulik (1977: replicated by several other studies) found that individuals can retain information from emotional memories more vividly than nonemotional memories. However, results suggest that while people may remember an emotional reaction vividly, the accuracy of the event may be in question (Sharot et al., 2004; Talarico & Rubin, 2003). Thus, for this study, it will be essential to measure the emotional toll of the stigma experienced on SNAP, not necessarily the exact event of stigma described, and consider accuracy of events for individuals who are no longer enrolled.

As discussed in the literature review, the experience of receiving SNAP benefits is situated within a wide range of personal and social contexts. Therefore, for both studies, I will analyze the following social determinants of health (demographic variables): race, gender, migrant status, types of stigma, age, and education level.

I have chosen the explanatory sequential mixed-methods design study because I need to understand what different types of stigma impact enrollment on SNAP before I can determine the social support mechanisms at play that can help or hurt how stigma is discussed and coped with. Without narrowing down what elements of stigma are impacting enrollment, interviewing broadly about stigma will potentially provide too wide a breadth of topics for meaningful analysis. Furthermore, understanding the factors that impact enrollment on SNAP is necessary to determine who needs to be interviewed to further describe the process of stigma as SNAP users, and how this identity is further impacted by the social support received. The study was approved by the Institutional Review Board (see appendix G for documentation). The process of identifying what stigma factors influence enrollment on SNAP will be determined in study 1.

Please note that the primary data collection for the research project occurred during the COVID-19, specifically in May 2020 for the survey data and June–August 2020 for the interview data; in this time there have also been several hurricanes that struck Louisiana. Because of the current disasters during the data collection process, some individuals may have been enrolled in D-SNAP.

SURVEY

Instruments

The first study will be to determine what social determinants of health (independent variables) impact enrollment on SNAP. Specifically, the different types of stigma and sources of stigma, and disclosure concerns, will be studied. Note all of the following studies were performed with participants who had been diagnosed with HIV; however, the questions have successfully been adapted to reflect SNAP membership and stigma based on the findings of the pilot studies.

To determine the different types of stigma, I will use a shortened instrument by Herek et al. that measures four different types of stigma experienced by individuals with HIV/AIDS: internalized, perceived, enacted, and vicarious. Based on a prior pilot study that combined Herek's types of stigma and parts of the DISC-12, the Cronbach α for the Herek's shortened scale which contained 17 questions was 0.96. I adapted the Herek scale to consist of three questions each addressing the different forms of stigma from SNAP enrollment: internalized stigma ($\alpha = 0.92$), perceived stigma ($\alpha = 0.92$), enacted stigma ($\alpha = 0.95$), and vicarious stigma ($\alpha = 0.92$) for a total of 12 questions. All types of stigma were found to significantly impact enrollment across several variables including education and migrant status in the third pilot study.

In the same pilot study, questions measuring friends, family, and poor stigma from the DISC-12 (Brohan et al., 2013) were used; the scale had an overall Cronbach α of 0.93. The questions measuring family stigma ($\alpha = 0.87$) and friend stigma ($\alpha = 0.93$) were acceptably reliable. Both stigma scales will be measured using a Likert scale format with 5 = strongly agree to 1 = strongly disagree. In other words, the higher the overall stigma score, the more reported stigma.

Next, to assess the impact of disclosure concerns, I used a scale created by Wright et al. (2007) adapted and shortened from Berger et al.'s (2001) larger instrument. I then adapted the Wright et al. (2007) scale to include questions related to stigma from SNAP enrollment. The Cronbach α for the Wright et al. study for disclosure concerns was 0.84. In the fourth pilot study, I found that disclosure concerns have the highest Cronbach α score for the Wright scale with 0.86. Furthermore, two questions will determine for whom the individuals have the highest disclosure concerns and ranking individuals based on how much disclosure concerns they have for each one.

In addition to the stigma measures, demographic questions (the social determinants of health) about race, age, migrant status, gender, generation of SNAP user, education, and total length enrolled on SNAP (the length enrolled will be reflected as months enrolled) will be asked. Finally, enrollment on SNAP will be measured with the dichotomous question, "Are you currently enrolled on SNAP? Yes or No." A copy of the measure is provided in appendix H.

Procedure

After performing an r^2 power analysis with 10 control variables (age, race, education, income, generation enrolled, and so on) and 10 test variables (the stigma variables and disclosure concerns), a power of 0.8 and a $p = 0.05$ the estimated sample size was 141. To ensure that I received at least that number, I recruited current or past SNAP recipients for my sample using LSU's Research Participation System, Amazon's MTurk, and individuals living in local parishes. Participants were compensated $0.40 for completing the survey on MTurk. A total of 385 participants were recruited, but once I removed participants who had never been enrolled on SNAP or had missing data, the sample size dropped to 295. After doing some initial testing, the sample size further decreased to 141, because participants had incomplete responses that impacted the logistic regression analysis. To enhance power, another sample was collected using MTurk, producing a total sample of 388 individuals. While several researchers have determined that using an MTurk sample is not representative of a generalized population (Woo et al., 2015; Brandon et al., 2014), Keith et al. (2016) note that using MTurk can be a helpful tool depending on the research project. For the current project, the MTurk sample had significantly more unemployed and part-time workers (Ross et al., 2010; Behrend et al., 2011). Overall, multiple studies indicate that using an MTurk sample does result in quality data (Clifford et al., 2015; Sheehan & Pittman, 2016).

To help remove some of the concerns with MTurk, I collected data from LSU's Research Participation System and individuals living in local parishes (counties) in Louisiana. Based on the prior pilot studies, no significant individual differences were found using different sources of data from SNAP participants. Because Qualtrics populates all of the results in a single data pool, it is impossible to determine which participant came from which sample without some type of identifier, which I did not use.

Once the data was compiled, I ran a variety of statistical analyses including pairwise correlation, Nested Logistic Regression, OLS regression, and ordered logistic regressions. After running the results, the data set was sent to an individual with statistical prowess in ordered logit to ensure that the "expert" found similar results before the questions for the interviews were formed. Based on these results, the questions for stigma and social support for the interviews of the explanatory mixed-methods design study were finalized. Furthermore, the demographics found in the survey data guided the selection of interview participants in an effort to have the participants who are interviewed correspond with those in study one in the hopes that some groups are not overrepresented in the interview data but not in the survey data.

INTERVIEW

For the interview portion of my study, a more phenomenological analysis or the analysis of everyday life from the viewpoint of the specific individual of the SNAP participants' experiences with stigma and social support and enrollment (Rogers, 1961) was used. I conducted semi-structured interviews, which were audio-recorded and transcribed.

Procedure

Using the findings from the survey instrument, I drafted an interview schedule (see appendix D) to perform in-depth interviews. Participants were recruited using three separate Facebook posts in which multiple individuals shared the posts. In addition to a Facebook blast, I also contacted the Office of Child Services and the LSU Graduate Association. After reaching out to these different platforms, I successfully interviewed 19 individuals (demographic information in next paragraph) who were either currently or had been enrolled in the past on SNAP. Participants are from a variety of parishes in Louisiana as well as different states, including Georgia, Ohio, New York, and New Mexico. Due to the nature of COVID, all individuals were interviewed using FaceTime, Zoom, or a cell phone call. I conducted the interviews because of my past experience with stigma from SNAP enrollment to help build rapport with the participants and become a vocal collaborator (Rapley, 2004).

At the beginning of the interview, I asked the consent form requirements, and once permission was given, I started recording interviewees' responses using Zoom; regardless of the medium used, no interviews were ever stored on my phone. Next, I asked the same demographic questions that had been completed for the survey instrument. Once the survey questions were completed, I began asking the questions from my interview schedule about experiences on SNAP with stigma and social support received. Though the projected time for the interview was about 30 minutes, five participants had shorter interviews of fewer than 30 minutes, and seven participants interviewed for over an hour (one was over two hours). I followed up with member checks to clarify information when needed. Member checks were used to help improve accuracy, credibility, and internal validity in my study (Birt et al., 2016). Sometimes if interviewees thought of more information, they reached out to me and shared.

Appendix C
Survey Demographics

A total of 388 participants were recruited using Amazon's MTurk engine (and were paid $0.40–0.50 for their participation), LSU's research participation system, and other local individuals enrolled in SNAP. To be considered for the study, all participants had to be a past or current member of the SNAP program. Participants who relied on SNAP benefits also reported living in a household size as ranging from one to more than six. Please note that not all of the categories equal to 388 participants; some chose not to respond to all of the questions. The average number of individuals who live in a household and benefit from SNAP aid is 2.67 (SD = 2.67). Of the participants, 294 were currently enrolled in the program, and length of SNAP enrollment ranged from 1 month to 28 years, for an average of 2.22 years (SD = 3.11) enrolled. The remainder of the sample had been enrolled in SNAP in the past ranging from 1 month to 10 years with an average of 1.44 years (SD = 1.42).

The sample consists of 253 individuals who reported as cisgender male (65.54%) and 133 reported as cisgender female (34.46%). The racial breakdown for participants consisted of 281 Caucasian participants (72.99%), African American or black 43 (11.17%), Hispanic 42 (10.91%), Asian 7 (1.82 %), Native American or Pacific Islander 9 (2.34%), and mixed racial background 3 (0.78%). Lastly, individuals reported the highest level of educational attainment as less than high school 6 (1.55%), high school graduate 30 (7.73%), some college 58 (14.95%), a two-year degree 77 (19.85%), a four-year degree 172 (44.33%), and professional degree 45 (11.60%). To determine what additional factors (social determinates) may impact enrollment, questions regarding migrant/temporary worker status, generation of immigrant, generation of SNAP receiver, and the type of SNAP received are asked.

Appendix C

As a reminder, a migrant or temporary worker is an individual who is in the United States on working visas such as the H-2A or H-2B or works only temporary jobs. The sample in the current study is one of the highest that I have recruited and it provides a unique diverse perspective. In the sample, 119 (31.23%) reported no migrant or temporary worker living in the household receiving SNAP benefits; 121 (31.76%) individuals stated they were the only migrant/temporary worker in the household; 77 (20.21%) individuals lived in a household in which their parents or guardians were migrant or temporary workers; 17 (4.46%) had significant others who were temporary/migrant workers; 3 (0.79%) reported another person living in the household as being a temporary or migrant worker; 32 (8.40%) individuals suggested that they were a temporary or migrant worker as well as a parent; and 12 (3.14%) had multiple members of the family as temporary or migrant workers including themselves, parents, and significant others.

In addition, of the individuals who reported a household member as well as themselves as a migrant or temporary worker, a high percentage also claimed they either were a first-generation immigrant or descended from immigrants. In the sample, 164 (43.73%) participants reported not being an immigrant or descended from immigrants, 102 (27.2%) were first-generation immigrants meaning they migrated from another country to the United States, 98 (26.13%) were born in the United States but had parents born in another country, and 11 (2.93%) had family members such as grandparents who were immigrants. The last two variables are specifically related to SNAP enrollment.

Individuals were asked in what generation of SNAP receivers they fit, specifically whether they are first-generation receivers, meaning they are the first in their family who has received benefits, second-generation receivers in which their parents also received benefits, or third-generation receivers in which both their parents and grandparents received benefits. In total, 169 (44.47%) reported being a first-generation SNAP receiver, 154 (40.53%) a second-generation recipient, and 57 (15%) a third-generation receiver. Having so many individuals who have prior family members with past SNAP experience may provide a unique viewpoint into how family dynamics may impact how an individual views stigma from the program. Next, I also asked participants what type of SNAP they had received in the past to determine how one may view stigma from regular SNAP benefits differently from disaster SNAP benefits. Most participants have been on regular SNAP only (272, 70.47%), but 58 (15.03%) had been enrolled in disaster SNAP benefits only. Lastly, 56 individuals (14.51%) reported being on both programs at some point.

Overall, the sample I have collected represents a more unique and diverse sample than I have received in previous pilot studies. This diversity can inform a discussion about intersectionality and stigma across different groups who are enrolled in SNAP.

Appendix D
Interview Schedule

THE EFFECTS OF STIGMA AND SOCIAL SUPPORT ON SNAP ENROLLMENT

Date and Location/Method

1. Opening Remarks
   a. Purpose of the study
   b. My prior history being a SNAP recipient
2. Informed Consent
   a. Permission to record
   b. Signed in person or verbal response
3. Main Questions
   a. Demographic questions
      i. Fill out the same demo questions as on the survey instrument.
      ii. Current enrollment question
         1. Are you currently or have been enrolled in the past?
            a. If you are no longer enrolled why did you leave?
   b. Total stigma questions
      i. Have you experienced being shamed, made fun of, bullied, or discriminated against for being a SNAP participant?
         1. Can you tell me about an event?
         2. How did you react to the event?
         3. Did it make you feel differently about your membership?
   c. Past consequences from disclosing SNAP enrollment stigma
      i. Have you ever "lost" members of your social circles after you told them you were enrolled in SNAP?
         1. Tell me about an example.
         2. Family? Friends? Coworkers?

                ii. Have individuals communicated less with you after telling them about your SNAP enrollment?
            d. Anticipated consequences from disclosing SNAP enrollment Stigma Questions—
                i. Now that I have asked specific questions about your experiences, how did this make you feel?
                    1. How did this event make you feel about yourself?
                    2. Do you feel the need to hide your enrollment from others?
                        a. Family? Friends? Coworkers?
                    3. Do you fear a negative reaction from your
                        a. Family? Friends? Coworkers? Because of your enrollment
            e. Social support and stigma questions
                i. Source of support
                    1. Do you talk about your SNAP enrollment?
                    2. If so with friends? Families? Others?
                        a. Do you discuss any shame or discrimination from being enrolled? With family, friends, others?
                        b. How does this support differ per person?
                    3. Who are you most concerned with disclosing your SNAP enrollment to?
                ii. Types of support
                    1. Do you receive any tangible, emotional, or informational when discussing the shame experienced?
                        a. Which of the above types of support affect you most positively when dealing with the shame from enrollment?
                        b. Can you provide examples of the different types of support that are used to help with the shame?
                        c. Does discussing about the shame help you cope with the damaging effects?
    4. Closing Remarks and Thanks
        a. How do you personally feel about SNAP as a whole?
        b. Do you intend to remain on SNAP longer? (This applies only to those individuals who are currently enrolled.)
        c. Thank you for everything today.

Appendix E
Procedure and Intercoder Reliability in Interview Data

Though the projected time for the interview was about 30 minutes, 5 participants had shorter interviews of fewer than 30 minutes, and 7 participants interviewed for over an hour (one was over two hours). I followed up with member checks to clarify information when needed. Member checks were used to help improve accuracy, credibility, and internal validity in my study (Birt et al., 2016). Sometimes if interviewees thought of more information, they reached out to me and shared.

The interviews were transcribed by the primary researcher, and the responses were compiled in Excel. After 15 participants, I started to notice repeating themes and responses, so I continued with 4 more interviews to make sure that I had reached saturation. During this process, I reached out to another researcher who has had experiences with the phenomenological and iterative process (Tracy, 2013; Rogers, 1961). I began analysis by reading and re-reading the data looking for themes. I then applied the constant comparison method to begin to refine codes or keywords in the data and compile an Excel spreadsheet to store the information. The first round of coding had 14 themes that had sufficient κ scores, but two variables—judgment and welfare abuse—had a κ of 0.60. The judgment theme consists of perceived, actual verbal, and actual nonverbal judgment, and includes statements about remarks or facial expressions because of one's SNAP enrollment. Welfare abuse theme includes the fear of being perceived as an abuser, having seen others abuse the program, and so on; this variable had an error in wording that caused issues with agreement. After re-norming on judgment and welfare abuse, all variables had a Cohen's κ of substantial or almost perfect agreement (Landis & Koch, 1977).

Appendix F
Limitations

As with any study, there are limitations or issues that were faced in the research process; this study is no different. The data collected used Amazon's MTurk engine prior to the COVID pandemic, whereas the data from the interviews was collected over the summer of 2020 in the midst of lockdowns. Thus, there may be some discrepancies in the stigmatizing view of SNAP that may have been influenced by COVID. Furthermore, COVID also made recruiting participants for interviews more difficult. My initial plan was to go to SNAP offices; however, at the time of data collection, many of these offices were closed, with most offices still closed (as of Fall 2020) to large numbers of participants coming in. These closures made it more difficult to go to the sources of SNAP participants in the different parishes, especially for areas that are harder hit with COVID numbers. Next, the social distancing guidelines made it impossible to get a face-to-face interview, especially with some participants voicing their concerns with meeting in person. Some of the responses in the interviews reflected the uncertainty and stigma caused by SNAP enrollment and COVID.

In addition to the intricacies relating to COVID and collecting data, it was also difficult to gather participants who were immigrants or migrant/temporary workers because of the international pandemic. While I was able to receive a few individuals in both categories, I would have liked more of a representation in the sample, but this is an area that will need further study.

Lastly, not related to COVID, the survey factor analysis indicated that all of the stigma variables from Herek et al. and DISC-12 loaded on 1 or 2 factors, which nulled many of my initial hypotheses. Prior pilot studies that I have conducted indicated distinct differences across all of the different types of stigma; however, in the current study, this was not the case. Though I am not sure of the cause in the current study, it warrants future research to determine why these different types of stigma did not come through, especially since in the interview process, respondents reported different levels of judgment. One potential issue could be that while these scales have been supported in prior studies, the Herek scale is an AIDS stigma scale and may not be interpreted as well when the instrument is modified to reflect stigma arising from other conditions or situations. Overall, while these limitations are present, I feel that they do not significantly weaken the results found in the current study and should lead to further research to adjust for these concerns as the pandemic lessens (hopefully), and more research and development of stigma scales are completed.

Appendix G
Survey Instrument

Q2 Are you currently enrolled or have been enrolled in the past (SNAP)? Yes or No

Q3 Are you currently enrolled in SNAP? Yes or No

Q4 How long have you been enrolled? Please specify months or years. For example, three months.

Q5 Why are you not currently enrolled in SNAP?

Q6 How long were you enrolled? Please specify months or years. For example, three months

Q7 What is your age? 17 or under or over 18? Please specify

Q8 What is your gender? Male, female, other

Q9 What is your race? White, Black or African-American, Hispanic, Asian, Native American or Pacific Islander, and Other

Q10 Select all that apply: Who in your household is a seasonal or migrant work who receives SNAP benefits? Yourself, Parents, Significant Other, Other, Not Applicable

Q11 What generation of immigrant are you? First (you immigrated from another country), Second (you were born in the United States, but parents are from another country), Other Not Applicable

Q12 What is your education? Less than high school, High school graduate, Some college, Two-year degree, Four-year degree, Professional degree, Doctorate

Q14 When compared to your close family, what generation of SNAP user are you? first generation (of my family we are the first to participate), second generation (my parents had SNAP as well), and third generation (my grandparents and parents had SNAP as well)

Q15 How many members in your household rely on SNAP benefits?

Q62 What type of SNAP benefits have you received? Regular SNAP benefits, Disaster SNAP benefits (storms, floods, COVID, etc.), or Both

START OF BLOCK: ENACTED STIGMA

Q54 Some people have reported negative experiences of shame and guilt because of their SNAP use. The following questions will ask you about your experiences with SNAP enrollment.
Q16 People have criticized me for my SNAP enrollment. (strongly disagree—strongly agree).
Q17 I have been mistreated by customers while using SNAP in a store. (strongly disagree—strongly agree.
Q18 I have received negative messages from people on social media about my SNAP enrollment (strongly disagree—strongly agree).
Q19 I have been called names for my enrollment on SNAP (user, doesn't work, stealing money, lazy, etc.) (strongly disagree—strongly agree)

END OF BLOCK: ENACTED STIGMA

Start of Block: Perceived Stigma

Q22 People view me differently because of my enrollment in SNAP (strongly disagree—strongly agree).
Q23 I see negative comments about SNAP users on social media, and think that the messages are directed at me (strongly disagree—strongly agree).
Q25 People view me differently at checkout in a store because of my SNAP enrollment (strongly disagree—strongly agree).

END OF BLOCK: PERCEIVED STIGMA

Start of Block: Vicarious Stigma

Q26 I have heard stories about people being called names for enrolling on SNAP (user, doesn't work, stealing money, lazy, etc.) (strongly disagree—strongly agree).
Q27 I know close friends who have been mistreated because of their enrollment on SNAP (strongly disagree—strongly agree).

Q28 I have family who have been mistreated because of their enrollment on SNAP (Parents, guardians, siblings, grandparents) (strongly disagree—strongly agree)

Q29 Other people I know have had bad experiences with other customers at the store over SNAP (strongly disagree—strongly agree).

END OF BLOCK: VICARIOUS STIGMA

Start of Block: Felt Normative Stigma

Q30 People in my local community (your town) disapprove of SNAP use (strongly disagree—strongly agree).

Q55 People in my state disapprove of SNAP use (strongly disagree—strongly agree).

Q31 People in society as a whole disapprove of SNAP use (strongly disagree—strongly agree).

END OF BLOCK: FELT NORMATIVE STIGMA

Start of Block: Internalized Stigma

Q32 I feel ashamed for my enrollment in SNAP (strongly disagree—strongly agree).

Q33 I have brought shame upon my family for enrolling in SNAP (strongly disagree—strongly agree).

Q34 I feel embarrassed for my enrollment on SNAP (strongly disagree—strongly agree).

END OF BLOCK: INTERNALIZED STIGMA

Start of Block: Family Stigma

Q35 I feel the need to hide my enrollment on SNAP from my family (strongly disagree—strongly agree).

Q36 I fear a negative reaction from family if I discuss my enrollment in SNAP (strongly disagree—strongly agree).

Q56 Because of my enrollment on SNAP I have lost family members (strongly disagree—strongly agree).

Q37 Because of my enrollment on SNAP family members communicate less with me (strongly disagree—strongly agree).

END OF BLOCK: FAMILY STIGMA

Start of Block: Friends Stigma

Q38 I feel the need to hide my enrollment on SNAP from my friends (strongly disagree—strongly agree).

Q39 I fear a negative reaction from friends if I discuss my enrollment in SNAP (strongly disagree—strongly agree).

Q40 Because of my enrollment on SNAP I have lost close friends (strongly disagree—strongly agree).

Q41 Because of my enrollment on SNAP close friends communicate less with me (strongly disagree—strongly agree).

END OF BLOCK: FRIENDS STIGMA

Start of Block: Workplace Stigma

Q42 I feel the need to hide my enrollment on SNAP from the people I work with (Coworkers, boss, associates, customers, etc.) (strongly disagree—strongly agree).

Q43 I fear a negative reaction from the people I work with (Coworkers, boss, associates, customers, etc.) when I discuss my enrollment in SNAP (strongly disagree—strongly agree).

Q57 Because of my enrollment on SNAP the people I work with (Coworkers, boss, associates, customers, etc.) communicate less with me (strongly disagree—strongly agree).

END OF BLOCK: WORKPLACE STIGMA

Start of Block: SES stigma

Q44 I feel people treat me differently because I am poor (strongly disagree—strongly agree).

Q59 I feel shame for being poor (strongly disagree—strongly agree).

Q60 I feel judged for being poor (strongly disagree—strongly agree).

END OF BLOCK: SES STIGMA

Start of Block: Discourse Concerns

Q49 I work hard to keep my SNAP status a secret (strongly disagree—strongly agree).

Q50 Telling someone I am a SNAP user is risky (strongly disagree—strongly agree).
Q51 I am very careful who I tell that I am a SNAP user (strongly disagree—strongly agree).
Q52 Who are you most concerned to tell that you are a SNAP user?
Q61 I fear disclosing to the following individuals because of my SNAP enrollment:

Close friends	(strongly disagree—strongly agree)
Friends	(strongly disagree—strongly agree)
Parents or guardians	(strongly disagree—strongly agree)
Close family	(please specify) (strongly disagree—strongly agree)
People you work with	(strongly disagree—strongly agree)
Strangers	(strongly disagree—strongly agree)
Significant Others	(strongly disagree—strongly agree)
Other	(strongly disagree—strongly agree)

END OF BLOCK: DISCOURSE CONCERNS

Start of Block: Enacted shame

Q20 What type of interaction with others leads to the most shame from your SNAP enrollment? Using the EBT card in a store, Disclosing your SNAP enrollment, Completing SNAP forms, How others view you, Other.

END OF BLOCK: ENACTED SHAME

Start of Block: Overall feeling of SNAP in general

Q53 Think of how you feel about the effectiveness of SNAP in general. On a scale from 1 to 5 how effective do you feel the program is worth providing you with income to purchase food?
(Scale of 1 to 5)

END OF BLOCK: OVERALL FEELING OF SNAP IN GENERAL

Bibliography

Aussenberg, R. (2018). Errors and fraud in the supplemental nutrition assistance program (SNAP). Congressional Research Service. https://fas.org/sgp/crs/misc/R45147.pdf

Bakhtin, M. M. (1986). *Speech genres and other late essays* (C. Emerson & M. Holquist, Eds.; V. McGee, Trans.). University of Texas Press.

Baxter, L., & Braithwaite, D. (2008). Chapter 26: Relational dialectics theory: Crafting meaning from competing discourses. In L. A. Baxter & D. O. Braithwaite (Eds.), *Engaging theories in interpersonal communication: Multiple perspectives* (2nd edition, pp. 349–362). SAGE Publications.

Behrend, T. S., Sharek, D. J., Meade, A. W., & Wiebe, E. N. (2011). The viability of crowdsourcing for survey research. *Behavioral Research Therapy, 43*, 1–14. doi:10.3758/s13428-011-0081-0

Berger, B., Ferrans, C., & Lashley, F. (2001). Measuring stigma in people with HIV: Psychometric assessment of the HIV stigma scale. *Research in Nursing & Health, 24*(6), 518–529. doi:10.1002/nur.10011

Birt, L., Scott, S., Cavers, D., Campbell, C., & Walter, F. (2016). Member checking: A tool to enhance trustworthiness or merely a not to validation? *Qualitative Health Research, 26*(13), 1802–1811. doi:10.1177/1049732316654870

Birtel, M., Wood, L., & Kempa, N. (2017). Stigma and social support in substance abuse: Implication for mental health and well-being. *Psychiatry Research, 252*, 1–8. doi:10.1016/j.psychres.2017.01.097

Brandon, D. M., Long, J. H., Loraas, T. M., Mueller-Phillips, J., & Vansant, B. (2014). Online instrument delivery and participant recruitment services: Emerging opportunities for behavioral accounting research. *Behavioral Research and Therapy, 26*, 1–23. doi:10.2308/bria-50651

Bresnahan, M., & Zhuang, J. (2016). Chapter 3: Stigma. In D. K. Kim & J. W. Dearing (Eds.), *Health communication research measures* (vol. 12, pp. 233–246). Peter Lang.

Brohan, E., Clement, S., Rose, D., Sartorius, N., Slade, M., & Thornicroft, G. (2013). Development and psychometric evaluation of the Discrimination and Stigma Scale (DISC). *Psychiatry Research, 208,* 33–40. doi:10.1016/j.psychres.2013.03.007

Bronfenbrenner, U. (1979). *The ecology of human development: Experiments by nature and design.* Harvard University Press.

Brown, R., & Kulik, J. (1977). Flashbulb memories. *Cognition, 5,* 73–99. doi:10.1016/0010-0277(77)90018-X

Browning, C., & Cagney, K. (2002). Neighborhood structural disadvantage, collective efficacy, and self-related health in a physical setting. *Journal of Health and Social Behavior, 43,* 383–399. doi:10.2307/3090233

Bruner, J. (1990). *Acts of meaning.* Harvard University Press.

Casale, M., Boyes, M., Pantelic, M., Toska, E., & Cluver, L. (2018). Suicidal thoughts and behavior among South African adolescents living with HIV can social support buffer the impact of stigma? *Journal of Affective Disorders, 245,* 82–90. doi:10.1016/j.jad.2018.10.102

Center for Immigration Studies. (2010). Immigration in the United States: A profile of America's foreign-born population. https://cis.org/Immigrants-United-States-Profile-Americas-ForeignBorn-Population

Clifford, S., Jewell, R., & Waggoner, P. (2015). Are samples drawn from Mechanical Turk valid for research on political ideology? *Research & Politics, 1,* 1–9. doi:10.1177/2053168015622072

Cooley, C. (1902). *Human nature and the social order.* Scribner.

Cooper, S., Campbell, G., Larance, B., Murnion, B., & Nielsen, S. (2018). Perceived stigma and social support in treatment for pharmaceutical opioid dependence. *Drug and Alcohol Review, 37,* 262–272. doi:10.1111/dar.12601

Crenshaw, K. (1989). Demarginalizing the intersection of race and sex: A black feminist critique of antidiscrimination doctrine, feminist theory and antiracist politics. *The University of Chicago Legal Forum, 1*(8), 139–167. doi:10.4324/9780429500480-5

Creswell, J., & Creswell, D. (2018). *Research design: Qualitative, quantitative, and mixed methods approaches* (5th edition). SAGE Publications.

Cucurullo, R. T. (2012). The special supplemental nutrition program for women, infants and children (WIC) and the supplemental nutrition assistance program (SNAP): Comparing policies and suggesting changes. *Journal of Food Law and Policy, 8*(257), 268–269.

Cutrona, C., & Suhr, J. (1992). Controllability of stressful events and satisfaction with spouse support behaviors. *Communication Research, 19*(2), 154–174. doi:10.1177/009365092019002002

Dilberto, M., & Schafer, M. (Spring 2018). Temporary foreign labor and sugar in Louisiana. *Louisiana Agriculture.* https://www.lsuagcenter.com/profiles/lbenedict/articles/page1528311878321

Domínguez, S., & Arford, T. (2010). It is all about who you know: Social capital and health in low-income communities. *Health Sociology Review, 19*(1), 114–129. doi:10.5172/hesr.2010.19.1.114

Eapen, D. (2016). *A qualitative description of pregnancy-related social support experiences of low-income mothers with low birth weight babies* [Doctoral Dissertation,

The University of Kansas]. KU Scholar Works. https://kuscholarworks.ku.edu/handle/1808/22491

Fisher, W. R. (1989). *Human communication as narration: Toward a philosophy of reason, value, and action*. University of South Carolina Press.

Fricke, H., Hughes, A., Schober, D., Pinard, C., Bertmann, F., Smith, T., & Yaroch, A. (2015). An examination of organizational and statewide needs to increase supplemental nutrition assistance program (SNAP) participation. *Journal of Hunger & Environmental Nutrition, 10,* 271–283. doi:10.1080/19320248.2015.1004217

Gans, H. (2011). The challenge of multigenerational poverty. *Challenge, 54*(1), 70–81. doi:10.2753/0577–5132540104

Goffman, E. (1963). *Stigma: Notes on the management of spoiled identity*. Simon & Schuster Inc.

Goldsmith, D. (2004). *Communicating social support*. Cambridge University Press.

Gregory, C., & Deb, P. (2015). Does SNAP improve your health? *Food Policy, 50,* 11–19. doi:10.1016/j.foodpol.2014.09.010

Gundersen, C., & Ziliak, J. (2015). Food insecurity and health outcomes. *Health Affairs, 34*(11), 1830–1839. doi:10.1377/hlthaff.2015.0645

Hair, J., Black, W., Babin, B., & Anderson, R. (2009). *Multivariate data analysis* (7th edition). Pearson Prentice Hall.

Harandi, T., Taghinasab, M., & Nayeri, T. (2017). The correlation of social support with mental health: A meta-analysis. *Electronic Physician, 9*(9), 5212–5222. doi:10.19082/5212

Harter, L., Japp, P., & Beck, C. (2005). Vital problematics about narratives theorizing about health and healing. In L. M. Harter, P. M. Japp & C. S. Beck (Eds.), *Narratives, health, and healing communication theory, research, and practice* (pp. 7–30). Erlbaum

Herek, G., Saha, S., & Burack, J. (2013). Stigma and psychological distress in people with HIV/AIDS. *Basic and Applied Social Psychology, 35,* 45–54. doi:10.1080/01973533.2012.746606

Higgins, T. (1987). Self-discrepancy: A theory relating self and affect. *Psychological Review, 94*(3), 319–340. doi:10.1037/0033-295X.94.3.319

House, J. (1981). *Work stress and social support*. Addison-Wesley.

Jensen, H., & Wilde, P. (2010). More than just food: The diverse effects of food assistance programs. *Agricultural & Applied Economics Association, 25*(3), 1–5.

Jones, E., Farina, A., Hastorf, A., Markus, H., Miller, D., & Scott, R. (1984). *Social stigma: The psychology of marked relationships*. Freeman.

Keith, M. G., & Harms, P. D. (2016). Is Mechanical Turk the answer to our sampling woes? *Industrial and Organizational Psychology, 9,* 162–167. doi:10.1017/iop.2015.130

Keith-Jennings, B., & Chaudry, R. (2018). Most working-age SNAP participants work, but often in unstable jobs. *Center for Budget and Policy Priorities, 1,* 1–22. https://www.cbpp.org/sites/default/files/atoms/files/3-15-18fa.pdf report

Kellas, J. (2008). Chapter 18: Narrative theories: Making sense of interpersonal communication. In L. A. Baxter & D. O. Braithwaite (Eds.), *Engaging theories in interpersonal communication: Multiple Perspectives* (2nd edition, pp. 241–254). SAGE Publications.

Kinsey, E., Oberle, M., Dupuis, R., Cannuscio, C., & Hillier, A. (Apr 2019). Food and financial coping strategies during the monthly supplemental nutrition assistance program cycle. *SSM Population Health, 7*, 1–8. doi:10.1016/j.ssmph.2019.100393

Kondrat, D., Sullivan, P., Barrett, B., Wilkins, B., & Beerbower, E. The mediating effect of social support on the relationship between the impact of experienced stigma and mental health. *Stigma and Health, 3*(4), 305–314. doi:10.1037/sah0000103

Korlagunta, K., Herman, J., Parker, S., & Payton, M. (2014). Factors within multiple socio-ecological model levels of influence affecting older SNAP participants' ability to grocery shop and prepare food. *Journal of Extension, 52*, 1–12.

Kunreuther, H., & Slovic, P. (1999, Summer). Coping with stigma: Challenges and opportunities. *Risk: Healthy, Safety, & Environment, 10*(3), 269–280.

Labov, W., & Waletsky, J. (1967). Narrative analysis: Oral versions of personal experience. In J. Helm (Ed.), *Essays on the verbal and visual arts: Proceedings of the 1966 annual spring meeting of the American Ethnological Society* (pp. 12–44). University of Washington Press.

Landis, J., & Koch, G. (1977). The measurement of observer agreement for categorical data. *Biometrics, 33*(1), 159–174.

Lehmann, C. (2019). Addressing social determinants of health. *PT in Motion, 11*(6), 28–39.

Link, B., & Phelan, J. (2001). Conceptualizing stigma. *Annual Review of Sociology, 27*, 363–385. doi:10.1146/annurev.soc.27.1.363

Liu, W., Sidhu, A., Beacom, A., & Valente, T. (2017). Social network theory. In Rössler, P., Hoffner, C., & Zoonen, L. (Eds.), *The International encyclopedia of media effects*. John Wiley & Sons.

Mandelbaum, J. (1987). Couples sharing stories. *Communication Quarterly, 35*(2), 144–170. doi:10.1080/01463378709369678

McLean, K., & Syed, M. (2016). Personal, master, and alternative narratives: An integrative framework for understanding identity development in context. *Human Development, 58*(6), 318–349. doi:10.1159/000445817

Meisenbach, R. (2010). Stigma management communication: A theory and agenda for applied research on how individuals manage moments of stigmatized identity. *Journal of Applied Communication Research, 38*(3), 268–292. doi:10.1080/00909882.2010.490841

Mohen, S., Gronenewegen, P., Volker, B., & Flap, H. (2011). Neighborhood social capital and individual health. *Social Science and Medicine, 72*, 660–667. doi:10.1016/j.socscimed.2010.12.004

Mokkarala, S., O'Brien, E., & Siegel, J. (2016). The relationship between shame and perceived origins of mental illness among South Asian and white American young adults. *Psychology, Health, & Medicine, 21*, 448–459. doi:10.1080/13548506.2015.1090615

Moseson, H., Mahanaimy, M., Dehlendorf, C., & Gerdts, C. (2019). "Society is, at the end of the day, still going to stigmatize you no matter which way": A qualitative study of the impact of stigma on social support during unintended pregnancy in early adulthood. *PLOS: One, 14*(5), 1–14. doi:10.1371/journal.pone.0217308

National Institute of Health. (2016). Health disparities. https://medlineplus.gov/healthdisparities.html

Nchako, C., & Cai, L. (2020). A closer look at who benefits from SNAP: State-by-state facts sheets. *Center on Budget and Policy Priorities, 1,* 1–2. https://www.cbpp.org/sites/default/files/atoms/files/snap_factsheet_louisiana.pdf

Nestle, M. (2019). The Supplemental Nutrition Assistance Program (SNAP): History, politics, and public health implications. *American Journal of Public Health, 109*(12), 1631–1635. doi:10.2105/AJPH.2019.305361

Ochs, E. (1997). Narrative. In T. van Dijk (Ed.), *Discourse as structure and process* (pp. 185–207). SAGE Publications.

Orbuch, T. L. (1997). People's accounts count: The sociology of accounts. *Annual Review of Sociology, 23,* 455–478. doi:10.1146/annurev.soc.23.1.455

Patton, S. (2012, May 11). The Ph.D. now comes with food stamps. *Chronicle of Higher Education,* p. A1. http://search.ebscohost.com.libezp.lib.lsu.edu/login.aspx?direct=true&db=f6h&AN=75194742&site=ehost-live&scope=site

Petronio, S. (2013). Brief status report on communication privacy management theory. *Journal of Family Communication, 13,* 6–14. doi:10.1080/15267431.2013.743426

Pinxten, W., & Lievens, J. (2014). The importance of economic, social, and cultural capital in understanding health inequalities: Using a Bourdieu-based approach in research on physical and mental health perceptions. *Sociology of Health & Illness, 36*(7), 1095–1110. doi:10.1111/1467-9566.12154

Psychology Today. (2020). *Psychologytoday.com.* Retrieved October 19, 2020, from https://www.psychologytoday.com/us/basics/embarrassment

Rapley, T. (2004). Interview. In C. Seale, G. Gobo, J. F. Gubrium, & D. Silverman (Eds.), *Qualitative research practice* (1st edition, pp. 15–33). SAGE Publications.

Reinius, M., Wettergren, L., Wiklander, M., Svedhem, V., Ekstrom, A., & Friksson, L. (2017). Development of a 12-item short version of the HIV stigma scale. *Health and Quality of Life Outcomes, 15*(115), 1–9. doi:10.1186/s12955-017-0691-z

Rogers, C. (1961). *On becoming a person: A therapist's view of psychotherapy.* Houghton Mifflin.

Ross, J., Zaldivar, A., Irani, L., & Tomlinson, B. (2010). *Who are the Turkers? Worker demographics in Amazon Mechanical Turk* [Paper presentation]. Association for Computing Machinery 28th ACM Conference on Human Factors in Computing Systems, Atlanta, GA, United States.

Roth, D. (2015). Food stamps: 1932-1977: From provisional and pilot programs to permanent policy. Economic Research Service, US Department of Agriculture.

Sayles, J., Hays, R., Sarkisian, C., Mahajan, A., Spritzer, K., & Cunningham, W. (2008). Development and psychometric assessment of a multidimensional measure of internalized HIV stigma in a sample of HIV-positive adults. *AIDS Behavior, 12,* 748–758. doi:10.1007/s10461-008-9375-3

Shankar, J., Ip, E., Khalema, E., Couture, J., Tan, S., Zulla, R., & Lam, G. (2013). Education as a social determinant of health: Issues facing indigenous and visible minority students in postsecondary education in western Canada. *International Journal of Environmental Research and Public Health, 10*(9), 3908–3929. doi:10.3390/ijerph10093908

Sharf, B., Harter, L., Yamasaki, J., &Haidet, P. (2011). Narrative turns epic: Continuing development in health narrative scholarship. In T. L. Thompson, R. Parrott, J. F. Nussbaum (Eds.), *The Routledge handbook of health communication* (2nd edition, pp. 36–51). Routledge: Taylor & Francis Group.

Sharot, T., Delgado, M., & Phelps, E. (2004). How emotions enhance the feeling of remembering. *Nature Neuroscience, 7,* 1376–1380. doi:10.1038/nn1353

Sheehan, K., & Pittman, M. (2016). *The academic's guide to using Amazon's Mechanical Turk: The HIT handbook for social science research.* Irving: Melvin & Leigh.

Smith R. (2007). Language of the lost: An explication of stigma communication. *Communication Theory, 17,* 462–485. doi:10.1111/j.1468-2885.2007.00307.x.

Talarico, J., & Rubin, D. (2004). Confidence, not consistency, characterizes flashbulb memories. *Psychological Science, 14,* 455–461. doi:10.1111/1467-9280.02453

Tracy, S. (2013). *Qualitative research methods: Collecting evidence, crafting analysis, communicating impact.* Wiley-Blackwell.

Uchino, B. (2004). The meaning and measurement of social support. In Alan Kazdin (Ed.), *Social support and physical health.* Yale University Press.

United Nations. (2019). More than meets the eye: Let's fight racism. https://www.un.org/en/letsfightracism/migrants.shtml

United States Census Bureau. (2019). Quickfacts Louisiana. https://www.census.gov/quickfacts/LA.

United States Department of Agriculture: Food and Nutrition Services. (2019). Characteristics of supplemental nutrition assistance program households: Fiscal year 2018. https://www.fns.usda.gov/snap/characteristics-supplemental-nutrition-assistance-program-households-fiscal-year-2018

United States Department of Agriculture: Food and Nutrition Services. (2019). Disaster supplemental nutrition assistance program (D-SNAP). https://www.disasterassistance.gov/get-assistance/forms-of-assistance/5769

United States Department of Agriculture" Food and Nutrition Services. (2020). SNAP data tables: National and/or state level monthly and/or annual data. https://www.fns.usda.gov/pd/supplemental-nutrition-assistance-program-snap

United States Department of Agriculture: Food and Nutrition Services. (2018). Supplemental nutrition assistance program (SNAP). https://www.fns.usda.gov/snap/eligibility

United States Department of Agriculture. (2019). Supplemental nutrition assistance program: Number of persons participating. https://fns-prod.azureedge.net/sites/default/files/pd/29SNAPcurrPP.pdf

United States Department of Agriculture. (2019). What is FNS Doing to Fight SNAP Fraud? https://www.fns.usda.gov/snap/integrity/fraud-FNS-fighting

United States Department of Labor. (2018). H-2A temporary agricultural program. https://www.foreignlaborcert.doleta.gov/h-2a.cfm.
United States Department of Labor (2018). H-2b temporary non-agricultural program. https://www.foreignlaborcert.doleta.gov/2015_H-2B_IFR.cfm.
United States News. (2020). Overview of Louisiana. https://www.usnews.com/news/best-states/louisiana
Vancil, A. (2008). Thanks, but no thanks: Potential food stamp recipients and why they decline the benefits. *Conference Papers--American Sociological Association*, *1*. http://search.ebscohost.com.libezp.lib.lsu.edu/login.aspx?direct=true&db=sih&AN=36955301&site=ehost-live&scope=site
Vaux, A. (1988). *Social support: Theory, research, and intervention*. Praeger.
Waxman, C. I. (1977). *The stigma of poverty: A critique of poverty theories and policies*. Pergamon Press, Inc.
Wellman, B. (1981). Applying network analysis to the study of support. In B. Gottlieb (Ed.), *Social networks and social support* (pp. 171–200). SAGE.
Wolfe, J., Kandra, J., Engdahl, L., & Shierholz, H. (2020). Domestic workers chartbook: A comprehensive look at the demographics, wages, benefits, and poverty rates of the professional who care for our family members and clean our homes. *Economic Policy Institute*, 1–65. https://files.epi.org/pdf/194214.pdf
Woo, S. E., Keith, M., & Thornton, M. A. (2015). Amazon mechanical turk for industrial and organizational psychology: Advantages, challenges, and practical recommendations. *Industrial and Organizational Psychology*, *8*, 171–179. doi:10.1017/iop.2015.21
World Health Organization. (2008). Social determinants of health: Key concepts. https://www.who.int/social_determinants/thecommission/finalreport/key_concepts/en/
World Population Review (2020). Welfare recipients by state 2020. https://worldpopulationreview.com/state-rankings/welfare-recipients-by-state
Wright, K., Naar-King, S., Lam, P., Templin, T., & Frey, M. (2007). Stigma scale revised: Reliability and validity of a brief measure of stigma for HIV1 youth. *Journal of Adolescent Health*, *40*, 1, 96–98. doi:10.1016/j.jadohealth.2006.08.001
Xiao, Z., Li, X., Qiao, S., Zhou, Y., & Shen, Z. (2018). Coping, social support, stigma, and gender difference among people living with HIV in Guangxi, China. *Psychology, Health, & Medicine*, *23*(1), 18–29. doi:10.1080/13548506.2017.1300671
Yen, S. T., Andrews, M., Chen, Z., & Eastwood, D. B. (2008). Food stamp program participation and food insecurity: An instrumental variables approach. *American Journal of Agricultural Economics*, *90*(1), 117–132. doi:10.1111/j.1467-8276.2007.01045.x

Index

Andrews, Margaret, 4
Arford, Tammi, 23

Bakhtin, Mikhail, 28
Barrett, Betty, 24
Baxter, Leslie, 28, 41
Beacom, Amanda, 22
Beck, Christina, 27, 40
Beerbower, Emily, 24
Behrend, Tara, 151
Berger, Barbara, 18, 20–21, 147, 150
Bertmann, F. M. W., 8, 20–21, 148
Birt, Linda, 152
Birtel, Michèle, 24
Boyes, Mark, 24
Braithwaite, Dawn, 28, 41
Brandon, Duane, 151
Bresnahan, Mary, 25
Brohan, Elaine, 18, 150
Bronfenbrenner, Urie, 7–8, 11–13, 33–34, 46, 58
Brown, Roger, 148
Browning, Christopher, 23
Bruner, Jerome, 26
Burack, Jeffery, 17–18, 20, 49–50, 52, 54–56, 77, 136, 141–42, 146–47, 149–50, 159–60

Cagney, Kathleen, 23
Cai, Lexin, 14

Campbell, Christine, 152
Campbell, Gabrielle, 24
Cannuscio, Carolyn, 5
Casale, Marisa, 24
Cavers, Debbie, 152
Center for Immigration Studies, 15
Chaudry, Raheem, 6
Chen, Zhuo, 4
Clement, Sarah, 18, 150
Clifford, Scott, 151
Cluver, Lucie, 24
Communication Privacy Management Theory, 25, 30–31, 33, 41, 44–47, 58, 98–99, 128, 136, 139–40
Cooley, Charles H., 9, 19, 21, 25, 36, 38, 46, 92
Cooper, Sasha, 24
Couture, Jennifer, 15
Crenshaw, Kimberly, 11
Creswell, David, 33, 148
Creswell, John, 33, 148
Cucurullo, Regina, 5
Cunningham, William, 21
Cutrona, Carolyn, 22

Deb, Partha, 4
Dehlendorf, Christine, 24
Delgado, Mauricio, 148
Dilberto, Michael, 14

disclosure concerns, 20–21, 27–28, 44, 46, 54, 99, 107, 109–10, 116, 131, 137, 141, 144, 147, 149–50; concern for disclosing SNAP enrollment to a specific person, 50–51, 59, 108, 114–15; generalized SNAP enrollment disclosure concerns, 21, 54
Dominguez, Silvia, 23
Dupuis, Roxanne, 5

Eapen, Doncy, 22
Eastwood, David, 4
education, 15–16, 29, 52, 57, 66, 78–80, 98, 102, 104, 109, 127, 132, 136–37, 149–50
Ekström, Anna, 21
Eriksson, Lars, 21

Farina, Amerigo, 17
Ferrans, Carol, 18, 20–21, 147, 150
Fisher, Walter, 26
Flap, Henk, 23
Frey, Maureen, 49, 55–56, 108, 136, 141, 144, 150
Fricke, H. E., 8, 20–21, 148

Gans, Herbert, 5–6
Gerdts, Caitlin, 24
Goffman, Erving, 4, 17–19, 21, 25, 29, 31, 36, 38, 46, 58, 75, 92
Goldsmith, Daena, 22–23
Gregory, Christian, 4
Groenewegen, Peter, 23
Gunderson, Craig, 4

Haidat, Paul, 27, 39
Harandi, Tayebeh, 4
Harms, Peter, 151
Harter, Lynn, 27, 39–40
Hastorf, Albert, 17
Hays, Ron, 21
Herek, Gregory, 17–18, 20, 49–50, 52, 54–56, 77, 136, 141–42, 146–47, 149–50, 159–60
Herman, Janice, 23

Higgins, Tory E., 19, 36, 38, 46, 92
Hillier, Amy, 5
Hughes, A. G., 8, 20–21, 148
hypotheses one through three, 18, 52, 154
hypothesis four, 18, 54, 76

immigrant status, 11–12, 14, 16, 34, 38, 52–53, 57, 75–79, 100–2, 104–5, 107–10, 131–32, 136, 154
intersectionality, 11, 38, 46, 49, 56, 58, 115, 117, 137, 140, 154
intertextuality, 27, 40–41
interview findings, 57; themes, 58–63 (avoiding discuss of SNAP enrollment, 58–60, 110–11, 113, 127; embarrassment, 36, 39–40, 58–59, 61, 65, 75, 80, 92–94, 96, 98–99, 114–15, 124–25, 128, 130, 137, 139; failure, 34, 36–40, 42, 46–47, 58–59, 63, 80, 92, 95–96, 98–99, 114, 127, 129–30, 137, 139; judgment, 30, 34, 37–41, 43, 58–59, 61, 80–85, 87, 92, 96–99, 115–20, 124–25, 127–30, 137, 139–40, 157; judging food choices, 38–39, 58–59, 62, 91, 94; laziness, 40, 58–59, 62, 92, 94–95, 114, 130, 137; necessity or survival, 58–59, 62, 65, 71, 74; political ideology, 34, 40, 59, 63, 135–36; race, 58–59, 62, 133–34; satisfaction/dissatisfaction with SNAP, 38–39, 58–60, 65, 68–70, 74; social support, 58–60, 113–14, 119–30; temporary enrollment, 58–59, 62, 73–74, 124; transitional state, 44, 58–59, 61, 65, 72–74, 124; welfare abuse, 35–36, 38–39, 43, 58–59, 61, 80, 85–87, 90, 157)
Ip, Eugene, 15
Irani, Lilly, 151

Japp, Phyllis, 27, 40
Jensen, Helen, 5
Jewell, Ryan, 151

Jones, Edward, 17

Keith, Melissa, 151
Keith-Jennings, Brynne, 6
Kellas, Jody, 26–27, 39
Kempa, Nancy, 24
Khalema, Ernest, 15
Kinsey, Eliza, 5
Koch, Gary, 157
Kondrat, David, 24
Korlagunta, Kiranmayi, 23
Kulik, James, 148
Kunreuther, Howard, 17

Labov, Williams, 26
Lam, Gavin, 15
Lam, Phebbe, 49, 55–56, 108, 136, 141, 144, 150
Landis, Richard, J., 157
Larance, Briony, 24
Lashley, Felissa, 18, 20–21, 147, 150
Lehmann, Christine, 8
Li, Xiaoming, 24
Lievens, John, 23
Link, Bruce, 25, 38
Liu, Wenlin, 22
Long, James, 151
looking glass self, 9, 19–21, 23, 25, 27, 31, 36, 92
Loraas, Tina, 151
Louisiana, 1, 13–16, 49, 67–68, 112, 146–47, 149, 151–52

Mahajan, Anish, 21
Mahanaimy, Moria, 24
Mandelbaum, Jerry, 27
Markus, Hazel, 17
Meade, Adam, 151
Mesienbach, Rebecca, 25–26, 36
migrant status, 8, 11–12, 14–16, 34, 38, 49, 51–53, 56–57, 75–80, 98, 100–2, 104–5, 107–10, 116, 131–32, 136–38, 140, 147, 149–50, 154
Miller, Dale, 17
Mohen, Sigrid, 23

Mokkarala, Sameera, 24
Moseson, Heidi, 24
Mueller, Jennifer, 151
Murnion, Bridin, 24

Naar-King, Sylvie, 49, 55–56, 108, 136, 141, 144, 150
narrative theory, 9, 25–26, 39, 46
National Institute of Health, 11
Nayeri, Tayebeh, 4
Nchako, Caitlin, 14
Nestle, Marion, 4
Nielsen, Suzanne, 24

Oberle, Megan, 5
O'Brien, Erin, 24
Ochs, Elinor, 26
Orbuch, Terri, 26

Pantelic, Marija, 24
Parker, Stephany, 23
Patton, Stacey, 15
Payton, Mark, 23
Petronio, Sandra, 30, 31, 44, 58
Phelan, Jo, 25, 38
Phelps, Elizabeth, 148
Pinard, C. A., 8, 20–21, 148
Pinxten, Wouter, 23
Pittman, Matthew, 151

Qiao, Shan, 24

race, 6, 8, 11–12, 14–16, 38, 42–43, 52, 58, 69, 75, 82, 94–95, 131, 136, 149–50
Rapley, Tim, 152
Reinius, Maria, 21
relational dialectics and the "chain of discourses", 9, 25, 28–29, 43–44, 46–47, 99, 129, 140
research question 1, 16, 52
research question 2, 18, 52, 117
research question 3, 18
research question 4, 54
research question 5.1, 24, 58–59

research question 5.2, 24, 59, 126
Rogers, Carl, 57, 151, 157
Rose, Diana, 18, 150
Ross, Joel, 151
Roth, Dennis, 5
Rubin, David, 148

Saha, Sona, 17–18, 20, 49–50, 52, 54–56, 77, 136, 141–42, 146–47, 149–50, 159–60
Sarkisian, Catherine, 21
Sartorius, Norman, 18, 150
Sayles, Jennifer, 21
Schafer, Mark, 14
Schober, D. J., 8, 20–21, 148
Scott, Robert, 17
Scott, Suzanne, 152
self-discrepancy theory, 19, 20, 36, 92
Shankar, Janki, 15
Sharek, David, 151
Sharf, Barbara, 27, 39
Sharot, Tali, 148
Sheehan, Kim, 151
Shen, Zhiyong, 24
Sidhu, Anupreet, 22
Siegel, Jason, 24
Slade, Mike, 18, 150
Slovic, Paul, 17
Smith, Rachel, 8, 20–21, 25, 38, 148
Smith, T. M., 8, 20–21, 148
social determinants of health, 4, 7–9, 11–13, 16, 52, 100, 110, 136, 138, 149
social ecological systems model, 7–8, 11–13, 16, 31, 33–34, 36, 46–47, 58, 136
social support, 3–4, 6, 8–9, 11–12, 14, 16, 21–25, 27–29, 33–34, 39–40, 47, 55, 64, 117, 131, 136–40, 145–46, 148–49, 151–52
spoiled identity, 9, 18–19, 21, 23–25, 29, 31, 36–39, 92
Spritzer, Karen, 21
stigma: anticipated consequences from disclosing SNAP enrollment, 18, 24, 36, 41, 50–51, 54–56, 59, 75, 98–99, 103–6, 109–10, 114–15, 130, 136, 143; past consequences from disclosing SNAP enrollment, 18, 24, 41, 45, 50–51, 54–56, 58–59, 75, 98–103, 105–6, 109–10, 114, 136–37, 143; SES stigma, 51, 54–55, 76, 78, 99–100, 104–5, 108, 144; theories of, 21, 25, 36; total stigma, 18, 24, 35, 41, 50–52, 54–56, 59, 75–79, 96, 98–103, 105–6, 110, 114, 116, 130, 132, 136–37, 142; types of, 17–18, 20, 24–25, 53–55, 58–59, 142, 146, 149–50, 159–60
Suhr, Julie, 22
Sullivan, Patrick, 24
supplemental nutrition assistance program (SNAP): D-SNAP, 5; fiscal information, 4; history of, 5; multigenerational poverty, 5, 6
survey findings, 49
Svedhem, Veronica, 21

Taghinasab, Maryam, 4
Talarico, Jennifer, 148
Tan, Shawn, 15
Templin, Thomas, 49, 55–56, 108, 136, 141, 144, 150
theory of stigma management communication, 25, 36–37, 81, 83–84, 98, 139
Thornicroft, Graham, 18, 150
Thornton, Meghan, 151
Tomlinson, Bill, 151
Toska, Elona, 24
Tracy, Sarah, 57, 157

Uchino, Bert, 22
United Nations, 15
United States Census Bureau, 14
United States Department of Agriculture, 4, 6, 14, 86, 90
United States Labor Department's Office of Foreign Labor Certification, 15

United States News, 15

Valentine, Thomas, 22
Vancil, Ashley, 8, 20–21, 148
Vansant, Brian, 151
Vaux, Alan, 22
Völker, Beate, 23

Waggoner, Philip, 151
Waletsky, Joshua, 26
Walter, Fiona, 152
Waxman, Chaim, 16
Wellman, Barry, 23
Wettergren, Lena, 21
Wiebe, Eric, 151
Wiklander, Maria, 21
Wilde, Parke, 5
Wilkins, Brittany, 24

Woo, Sang E., 151
Wood, Lisa, 24
World Population Review, 13
Wright, Kathryn, 49, 55–56, 108, 136, 141, 144, 150

Xiao, Zhiwen, 24

Yamasaki, Jill, 27, 39
Yaroch, A. L., 8, 20–21, 148
Yen, Steven, 4

Zaldivar, Andrew, 151
Zhou, Yuejiao, 24
Zhuang, Jie, 25
Ziliak, James, 4
Zulla, Rosslynn, 15

About the Author

Dr. Laura Blount Carper earned her Ph.D. from Louisiana State University in Communication Studies, with a focus on interpersonal communication, specifically on health and risk communication. This project is the culmination of years of research on her passion, welfare assistance programs, specifically SNAP. She is passionate about studying the voices of individuals who live in poverty and how welfare assistance programs, such as SNAP and WIC, are stigmatizing. In addition to her work with stigma and SNAP, she studies infertility/pregnancy and stigma, vaccination rates, and social support. She hopes to extend her research into stigma of eating disorders, miscarriage and bereavement, and many others. She is also a proud mom of two, and lives in Louisiana. She is currently an instructor at Louisiana Tech University.

www.ingramcontent.com/pod-product-compliance
Lightning Source LLC
Chambersburg PA
CBHW021356300426
44114CB00012B/1247